# INTEGRATIVE FACIAL CUPPING

## Lymphatic drainage and face-lifting protocols

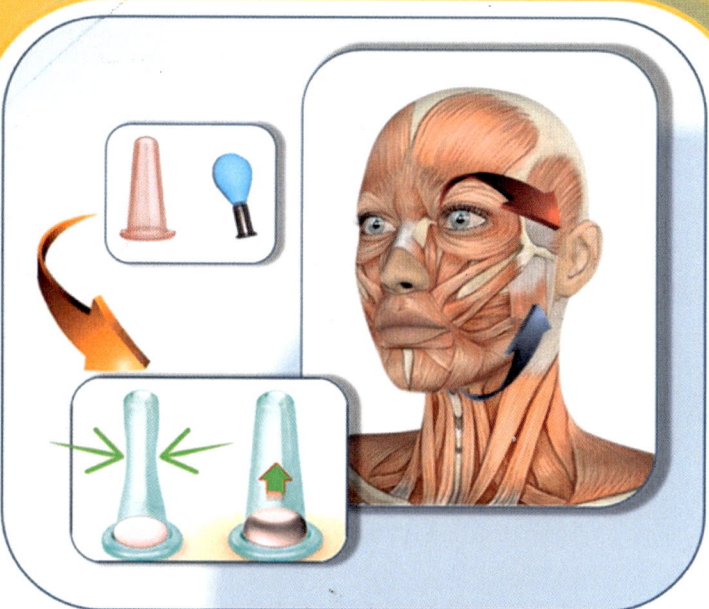

...QUICK LEARNING...

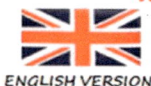
ENGLISH VERSION

Dr. Carlos Paulo

Dear reader,

I hope you will enjoy reading this book.

For this, I searched in the annals of plastic surgery, think about the order of protocols and review the anatomy. The lymphatic system has not said its last word ...

This book is an original text. Thank you to respect copyright.

Kind regards, Dr. Carlos Paulo.

# TABLE OF CONTENTS

*TABLE OF CONTENTS ................................................................................. 3*
   General introduction ............................................................................ 7
   About the author ................................................................................... 8

*PART 1 - BASIC LYMPHATIC DRAINAGE ............................................... 10*
   Presentation ........................................................................................ 10
   Benefits of facial cupping ................................................................... 11
   Indications of facial cupping .............................................................. 12
   Contre indications .............................................................................. 12
   Questions about facial cupping ......................................................... 12
      Facial cupping? ................................................................................ 12
      Objectives of facial cupping ........................................................... 13
      Different suction cups applications ............................................... 13
      Bruising with cups? ........................................................................ 13
      How does cupping work? ............................................................... 14
      Cupping and lymphatic drainage ................................................... 14
      Application protocol ...................................................................... 14
      Immediate effects and precautions ............................................... 14
      What types of cups? ....................................................................... 15
      Disclosure ....................................................................................... 15
   General cupping protocol .................................................................. 16
      Basic technique .............................................................................. 16
      Basic movements ........................................................................... 16
   Specific cupping protocol .................................................................. 18
      *Venus – Star* protocol .................................................................. 18
         First step: a trip to Venus ......................................................... 18
         Second step: a trip to a star ..................................................... 18
      Protocol details .............................................................................. 19
         Eight points chronology ........................................................... 19
         Eight points movements .......................................................... 20

## PART 2 - COMPLEMENTARY COURSE ..................................................23

**Introduction** ........................................................................................23

**Veno-lymphatic drainage** ...............................................................23
- Position of lymphatic nodes .................................................................23
- Lymphatic and venous drainage ..........................................................24

**With or without valves?** .................................................................25
- General presentation of the lymphatic system ...................................25
- Lymphatic capillaries without valves ...................................................26
- Lymphatic vessels with valves .............................................................26

**Skin and lymphatic capillaries** ......................................................27

**Additional movements for neck and face** ..................................29
- Posterior region of the neck ................................................................29
- Long journey movement ......................................................................29

**Additional movements for eyes area** .........................................31
- Drainage direction in the eyelid area...................................................31
- Other observations on eyelid drainage ...............................................32
- Eyelid, a particular crossroads of drainage ........................................32

**Puffiness drainage** ...........................................................................33
- Understanding ......................................................................................33
- Surface anatomy and drainage ...........................................................33

**Additional movements for submandibular area** .....................35

**Remarks for additional movements** ..........................................37

**Nervous stimulation of the face** .................................................39

**Nervous stimulation between face and back/neck** ................40
- Example of splenius muscles ..............................................................40
  - Mobile suction step .........................................................................41
  - fixed suction step ............................................................................42
  - notes .................................................................................................43

## PART 3 - FACE-LIFTING AND COMESTIC APPLICATIONS ......................45

**Introduction** ........................................................................................45

**Face-lifting protocols** ......................................................................45
- Difference between lymphatic drainage and face-lifting ..................45

How long to try to be less rided?........................................................................46
Gradual intensity of aspiration ...........................................................................46

## Cheek protocol ........................................................................................47
Introduction .........................................................................................................47
Chronology..........................................................................................................47
    First step: The upward orientation ................................................................47
    Second step: Fixed cups .................................................................................47
    Second step: Variant ......................................................................................48
Illustration...........................................................................................................48
    First step .......................................................................................................49
    Second step...................................................................................................49
Reasoning ...........................................................................................................50
    First step .......................................................................................................50
    Second step...................................................................................................50
Conclusion ..........................................................................................................51

## Rejuvenation protocol ............................................................................52
Introduction .........................................................................................................52
Chronology..........................................................................................................52
    First step: Mobile ..........................................................................................52
    Second step: Fixe ..........................................................................................53
Illustration...........................................................................................................53
    First step: Mobile ..........................................................................................54
    Second step: Fixe ..........................................................................................54

## Three forces protocol ............................................................................55
Introduction .........................................................................................................55
Chronology..........................................................................................................55
    First step: Rotation ........................................................................................55
    Second step: Smoothing ................................................................................56
    Third step: Compression ................................................................................56
Illustration...........................................................................................................56
    First step: Rotation ........................................................................................56
    Second step: Smoothing ................................................................................57
    Third step: Compression ................................................................................58
Reasonning .........................................................................................................58
    First step .......................................................................................................58
    Second step...................................................................................................59
    Third step .....................................................................................................59

## *PART 4 - COMPLEMENTARY METHODS..................................................61*

# Introduction .................................................................................................. 61
# Which oil can i use? ..................................................................................... 62
## The various oils possible ............................................................................ 62
## Why olive oil? .......................................................................................... 62
# Jala neti ..................................................................................................... 63
## Description ............................................................................................. 63
### Material ................................................................................................ 63
### Technique ............................................................................................. 63
### Reasoning ............................................................................................. 64
# Oil therapy in the mouth ............................................................................. 65
## Description ............................................................................................. 65
### Material ................................................................................................ 65
### Technique ............................................................................................. 65
### Reasoning ............................................................................................. 65
# Drainage gland of mebomian ...................................................................... 66
## Description ............................................................................................. 66
### Material ................................................................................................ 66
### Technique ............................................................................................. 66
### Reasoning ............................................................................................. 67
# *REFERENCES ............................................................................................. 68*

# General Introduction

It is a simple and effective technique. The action of the suction cups acts on the different depths of the skin. Muscles, fascia and all vascular and nerve structures are stimulated. The facial cupping will have a manual lymphatic drainage (MLD) effect and muscle relaxation. There will also be a "plumping" (repulpant) effect with myofascial decompression. Also, there will be a "colouring" effect because the blood is attracted under the skin using a small silicone suction cup.

So the keywords of facial cupping are drainage, lifting, muscle release and toning! The cupping facial takes care of the whole face and the surrounding areas (face, neck and "decollete").

The cupping facial of this book is not based on Chinese medicine. It is based on the anatomical knowledge of the muscles and lifting concepts that are found in other manual massage. By its physiological effect, cupping facial provides many reliefs.

**The first part,** insists on lymphatic drainage. It wants to be autonomous and practical for anyone with little anatomical knowledge. The goal is to reach a practice of 15 to 20 minutes to do 2 to 3 per week (like a jogging). It has two essential stages: the drainage of the neck towards the triangle of Venus (Trip to Venus!) and the drainage of the face (Trip to a star!). *Try the Venus – Star protocol!*

**The second part,** is a deepening of the knowledge of the first part on lymphatic drainage, and we will see that sometimes it goes beyond the cosmetic field. Complementary movements are added and can be applied for the *"Venus-Star"* protocol, depending on your experience. There will also be close links between the lymphatic system and the venous system.

**The third part,** is an application of suction cups for the rejuvenation and treatment of facial wrinkles. Three protocols will be presented in relation with the mechanical properties of the skin and the aging of the face. A protocol will be presented according to the work of specialist Mr. Chirali. The protocol of this author is based in part on Chinese medicine. The first part of this book on lymphatic drainage could be included in facial rejuvenation protocols. *Try three rejuvenation protocols!*

**The fourth part,** explains three tips or methods that are included in the concept of integrative facial cupping. In fact, the face is a functional unit included in the whole of the cephalic extremity (the head). The face is a structure plated on a hollow sphere that is called the head. So cleaning the mouth, nasal cavities, massage of the Meibomian glands are techniques included in this concept.

## ABOUT THE AUTHOR

Dr. Paulo Carlos, general practitioner living in southern Spain.

French medical formation, he is moving towards alternative medicine and cupping therapy.

E.mail contact: paulo.cupping@gmail.com

# Integrative Facial Cupping Part 1

## Basic lymphatic drainage

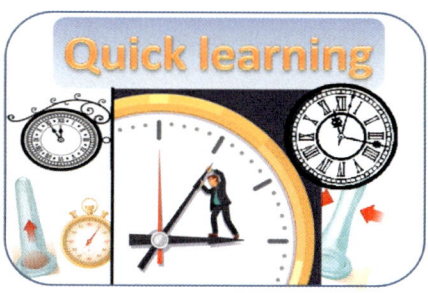

## Venus - Star protocol

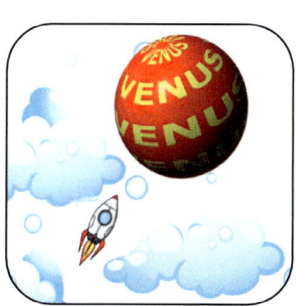
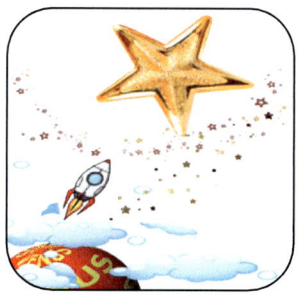

# PART 1 - BASIC LYMPHATIC DRAINAGE

## PRESENTATION

It is a superficial and profound technique at the same time.

- Superficial

Anti-wrinkles effect by compression and decompression of the skin.
Toning and colouring effect by hyperemia physiology with cups.

- Deep

Veno-lymphatic drainage effect which is a slow speed system.
Vascularisation effect by the arteries which is a fast speed system.
Myofascial liberation effect and evacuation of lactic acid and impurities.

It is a variable speed technique. Depending on the application speed of the suction cups, different effects can be obtained. The slow speed is draining (edema, toxins) and the fast speed is stimulating (collagen).

The use of silicone suction cups or small suction cups allows to adapt to the delicacy of the skin of the face. It can be complementary to other techniques because it is physiological.

From the historical point of view, the use of suction cups is very old and is found in all countries (there are more than 5000 years in China). In the countryside, it is often a popular remedy. Currently, sportsmen, celebrities are very interested in body cupping or facial cupping. With the advancement of technology, the development of silicone suction cups allows more ease of application for the face and fragile areas (inner limbs). This first part, insists on lymphatic drainage.

# BENEFITS OF FACIAL CUPPING

### Reduction of wrinkles

This is one of the most wanted effects in facial cupping. Decrease of the bags (puffiness) under the eyes...

### Healing after surgery

Cups are well-known for helping to have good healing (depressotherapy with highly advanced devices). Scar massage is inspired by certain progressive techniques of myofascial liberation.

### Activation of the inmune system

By increasing lymphatic drainage and vascularisation. There are many studies that demonstrate improvement regarding autoinmune diseases. A functioning organ with good drainage and good blood supply has a better chance of defending itself from the inmune point of view.

### Relaxation

The effect of reflexotherapy is obvious, it induces a relaxation like many massages.

### Decongesting effect

This is one of the important effects of cupping massage and facial cupping. The cup draws blood under the skin. It allows "moving" toxins and stagnant molecules. The face and neck are drained by the axillary lymph nodes.

### Other benefits

We do not count the other benefits! They are very numerous! Nutrient supply, oxygenation. From the point of view of Chinese medicine, it unblocks the energy channels. Improvement of sinusitis problems and paralysis of the facial nerve. Increased absorption of skin care products...

## INDICATIONS OF FACIAL CUPPING

Cupping facial indications come from all the benefits. These are all the problems of edemas, venous, overload, sinusitis, pain...Depending on the therapist's experience and the condition of the patient, the cupping session may be directed towards lymphatic drainage or a more targeted action on the muscle. This first part, insists on lymphatic drainage. Overload, sinusitis, pain...

## CONTRE INDICATIONS

We must adapt to the patient and his skin. Find out if the patient has cutaneous cancer, autoinmune skin disease, venous thrombosis. If exposure to the sun is too important, make sure not to stimulate the skin with cupping too much. Do not use facial cupping when an infection is present. Avoid if possible to massage too hard on moles.

## QUESTIONS ABOUT FACIAL CUPPING

### FACIAL CUPPING?

It is the application of silicone suction cups or small suction cups, adapted to allow a lifting of the skin and a detachment of the under-skin. Its purpose can be therapeutic as well as aesthetic. It can have "anti-aging" effects against environmental aggressions (sun, polluting particles, etc.). Cupping facial is oriented towards all natural procedures, without chemicals. It uses a dermoprotective massage oil, the most organic possible (Jojoba or others).

## OBJECTIVES OF FACIAL CUPPING

By the many benefits of cupping, several objectives can be proposed.

- The anti-wrinkle effect is one of the most sought after by its plumping action and collagen stimulation. This anti-wrinkle effect can be combined with contraction massage and stretching of the muscles. The anti-wrinkle effect is also achieved by adapting to the anatomy of the muscles of the face.

- The suction effect of suction cups removes impurities from the skin and makes drainage to the ganglia.

- The effect of tissue detachment allows a release of fascia and reduces muscle contractures.

- The additional blood supply to the skin also allows its regeneration, nutrition and intake of defense cells (such as white blood cells).

## DIFFERENT SUCTION CUPS APPLICATIONS

The facial cupping is mostly done with movable suction cups to avoid too strong red marks on the face. But you can also use fixed suction cups to firm and tone some areas of the face. The mobile suction cups stimulate the collagen and make a movement according to the anatomy of the muscle. In-depth stimulation of the skin's muscles is one of the main features of cupping. Lymphatic drainage is also possible as evidenced by this document.

## BRUISING WITH CUPS?

Normally, the cupping facial does not produce bruises on the face because there is no trauma. In addition, this is done with small suction cups limiting accidents by too much suction. In the bruise, a vein or artery can be harmed, letting blood escape to the skin tissue such as during a boxing match. This is not the case with the cupping facial.

## HOW DOES CUPPING WORK?

When the vacuum is created inside the cup, we have an increase in local circulation under the skin. This can even create a "Hyperemia". Indeed, the fascia under the skin heats up, separates (due to a three-dimensional collagen system in this region). Many blockages disappear (some say energetic), the stagnant lymph moves. The blood supply also brings a moisturizing element to the skin and oxygen from the red blood cells.

## CUPPING AND LYMPHATIC DRAINAGE

Most manual lymphatic drainages act first in compression, it is not easy. They are carried out slowly and at "low" pressure. The cupping massage is done in part in reverse: in "decompression". This decompression also allows the opening of the lymphatic capillaries located under the skin. In addition, the suction cup with its edges in contact on the skin also acts in compression! It is necessary to take care of the direction of application of the suction cup that is to say not to make movement of back and forth. It is necessary to massage in the direction of the flow of the lymphatic capillary. The application of a heat source on the skin will facilitate drainage from the vascular and lymphatic points of view.

## APPLICATION PROTOCOL

The suction cups apply in static and dynamics. The suction cups are designed to produce a gentle suction pressure. They are applied to the well-oiled skin to slide them. The large suction cup will be used for larger areas and smaller for smaller areas (or to work a specific area).

## IMMEDIATE EFFECTS AND PRECAUTIONS

The lymphatic system is an important waste disposal system. After many stages, the lymph reaches the level of the cardiovascular system (into the heart!). Please hydrate yourself because it is a fluid system. When the toxins move in the lymphatic veins, the body will feel lighter. Paradoxically, you may feel a little nauseated, with a feeling of fog. This is because the body tries to eliminate toxins. Also, this is because the toxins have moved. Once you have crossed this path, you will feel better and much more relaxed with better sleep.

The whole area O.R.L (**ears, nose and larynx**) will be unloaded, which will improve the problems of sinusitis, headaches. The effect on wrinkles will be evident before and after the session. You can even take a picture before and after to compare! It is also one of the effects most sought after by women in the cupping facial.

## WHAT TYPES OF CUPS?

One of the important features is the use of small cupping because the skin of the face is fine. The skin of the eyelids is the thinnest (less than 1 mm). By their low depression, they adapt to the delicacy of the face.

- For lymphatic drainage of the face, small rubber or silicone suction cups are ideal, as we will see in this book.
- Plastic suction cups can be used for larger areas and during the facial rejuvenation protocol with a larger blood supply, which will be discussed later.
- Sometimes fixed plastic suction cups are used, according to the experience of the practitioner. If we do not want red marks, we must leave them in place for a maximum of 2 minutes. Everything depends on the patient, his skin, his willing to participate and acceptance of some temporary red marks, (especially in the cosmetic field).

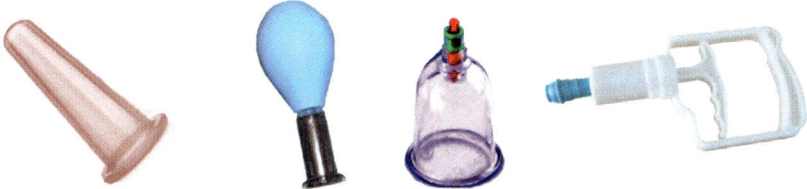

## DISCLOSURE

Do not use facial cupping when an infection is present. Indeed, lymphatic drainage can diffuse the microbes present in the ganglia. *If in doubt about the condition of the face or skin, consult a doctor*. It is a hygienic, anti-wrinkle and detoxifying method of care. The therapeutic effects are due to the healthy physiological participation of the suction cups. Cupping facial can accelerate healing processes, it is a complementary treatment. If you have the opportunity to use glass or plastic suction cups, please check the rims (see if they are smooth, to avoid injury).

# GENERAL CUPPING PROTOCOL

### BASIC TECHNIQUE

- Usually, 15 to 20 minutes and can be a complementary or autonomous treatment (if you want to work in depth, on muscle relaxation, the session can last longer).
- The silicone suction cups have a gentle suction and are painless. There should be no red mark on the skin. However, some patients have red skin very quickly.
- In general, the repetition of the movement is 3 times in each zone. Alternating on each side of the body. But we can go up to 50 times, if we have time. This allows you to work more deeply.
- The speed of movement produces different therapeutic effects:
    - Slow speed produces a greater drainage effect and reduces bags (puffiness) under the eyes.
    - Fast speed produces a stimulating effect on collagen, circulation and tonicity.
- This protocol is composed of two important chronological and anatomical steps (as we will see in the following paragraph.
- Adapt well to the patient's skin, depending on the age and health of the patient.

### BASIC MOVEMENTS

- The lines and arrows represent the direction of the suction cup's movement.
- **The stars** represent the zone of "static" cups. Do not slide on these areas (or really less).
- The yellow circles represent the possibility of making spirals.

For a drainage effect, first begin under the chin to unload the lymphatic channels (or clavicular region). The technique should be performed 3-5 times in each zone (see even up to 50 slow spiral movements).

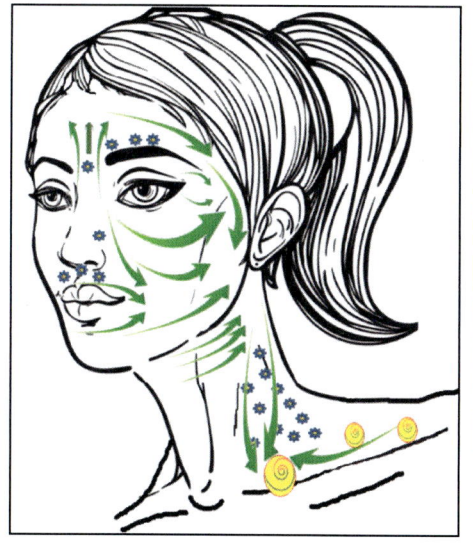 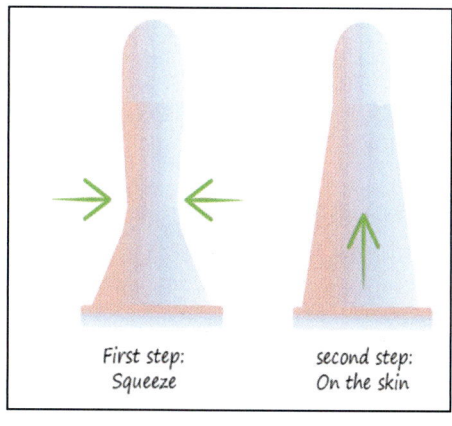

The direction of the suction cup's movement spiral, static and dynamic movement.

Squeeze the suction cup to expel the air inside. Then put it on the skin for the massage.

# Specific cupping protocol

## Venus – Star protocol

### First step: a trip to Venus

If we were to say a key word for the drainage of the face and neck, it is "Venus" or more precisely the region of the triangle of Venus. This is where we will "direct" all the lymph from the upper body and therefore the face. The lower parts of the head (neck and collarbone area) are first drained before draining the face.

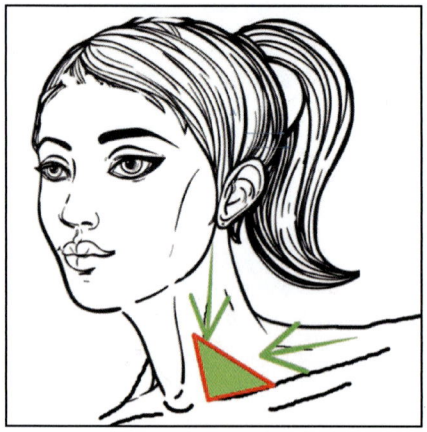

The Venus triangle:
Lymph convergence zone

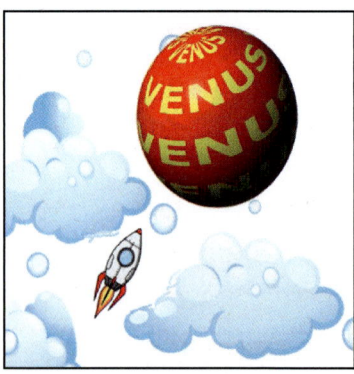

First step:
Facial cupping is a trip to Venus

### Second step: a trip to a star

Another key word is the word "star". Indeed, when one does not know well the anatomy of the lymph nodes, it is useful to represent the area of convergence of the lymphatic vessels in the form of a star. After draining in first steps, the lower regions below the face towards Venus. It will drain the lymph of the face to this "5-pointed star" representing the main lymphatics draining it. Then you can combine the two steps: Start from one place of the face, go through the star and return to Venus. It's a very simple drainage! It's objective "Venus"!

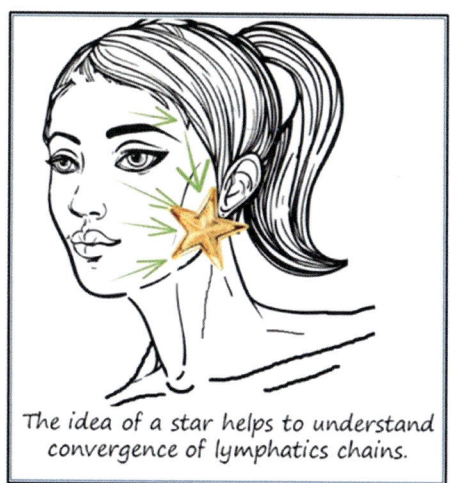
The idea of a star helps to understand convergence of lymphatics chains.

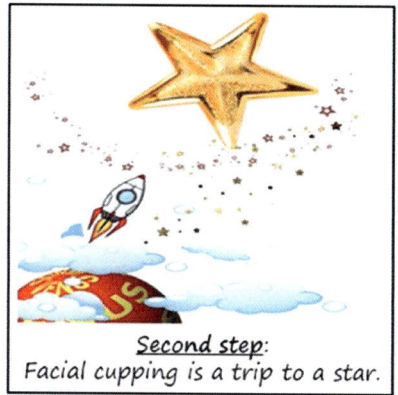
*Second step*:
Facial cupping is a trip to a star.

## PROTOCOL DETAILS

### EIGHT POINTS CHRONOLOGY

We wrote a small chronology in 8 points to start. It is a general plan that will then allow you according to your experience, to go further. Recall, the rhythm must be very soft, slow with little pressure. That's why we use silicone suction cups. Above all, do not fail to do the first phase, the trip to "Venus" before making the trip to "the star". Then, as mentioned above, you can combine the two steps: Start from one place of the face, go through the star and return to Venus. That is to say follow the downward direction of physiological lymphatic drainage.

### Eight points movements

**A** – Cleaning the skin and applying the massage oil.

**B** – Going to Venus:

Just like in classic manual drainage, let's start with the "décolleté". The goal is to release the lower lymph node regions (relative to the head). Start with the sternum area, and then go to the hollow of the supraclavicular regions (above the clavicles). Make also a movement of the sucker going from the shoulder to the region of the triangle of Venus. Repeat 3 to 5 times each movement. For these larger areas, you can take a big suction cup. The repetition number of 3 to 5 times is an average. However, it is a hinge area where all the lymph will come together, so it will be useful to do more than 50 suction spiral movements associated with a small pumping. The goal is to ensure a good evacuation of the lymph. If you have time, you can do it with your hands as well.

**C** – Going to Venus via the star:

Then, for the following areas, take a small suction cup. Start with the area below the chin, and gradually descend to the clavicle area. The goal is to follow the direction of the lymphatics, as they move downwards towards the clavicle and then the heart. Repeat 3 to 5 times each movement. Be careful; do not go up with the cup to the jaw, because the goal is to produce a movement of descent of the lymph. Eventually, you can do it at the end of the session.

**D** – Short decompression technique by zone:

This is a brief installation (1 to 2 seconds) of the suction cup and removes each time. The goal is to make a kind of localized "pumping". This is stimulating and aims to open the "lymphatic nodes" that run through the entire neck area.

**E** – Moving the suction cup from the chin area to the lateral edge of the jaw (i.e. to the ears). Then redo again, the technique (D) of short decompression by zone at the neck. You can also make descending movements of the suction cup.

F – Repeat the technique (D) of short decompression by the area around the lips and eyes (see diagram). Continue by sliding the suction cup on the cheek or on the temples, then finish towards the neck area. When arriving at the neck, do the brief decompression technique. The eyes and lips are highly charged areas both in terms of emotions and in the appearance of wrinkles. It must therefore be unburdened; at least from the lymphatic point of view (We will see later in this book, that the lymphatic drainage of the eyelids has some peculiarities).

G – Finish lymphatic drainage by the area of the root of the nose. Slide the suction cup "vertically" (or slightly obliquely, because the muscle bundles are not really vertical). Vertically, that is to say, eyes towards the scalp.

H – Slide the suction cup "horizontally" on the forehead. Then continue down to the neck.

Conclusion: This is a general plan that aims to be practical for a session of 15 to 20 minutes. We can go further; taking the books of the lymphatic drainage, and insisting on more specific areas. The most important thing is to be able to drain at the neck, so that the waste can be eliminated. Some Chinese masters of long life gymnastics have also insisted on the massage of the neck area. Indeed, the brain also needs to be drained just as much as the face! And that goes through the neck. Then, take all your time for the face.

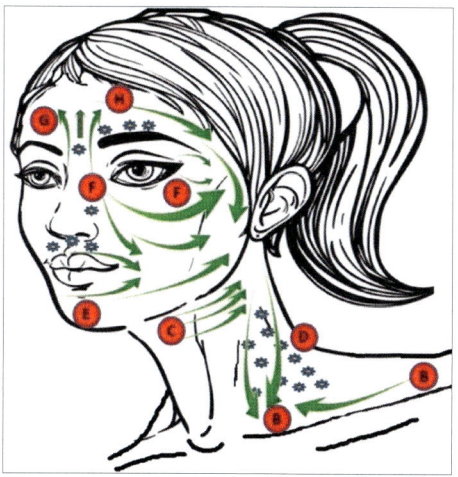

# Integrative Facial Cupping Part 2

## Complementary course of lymphatic drainage with cupping

### Let's go further !

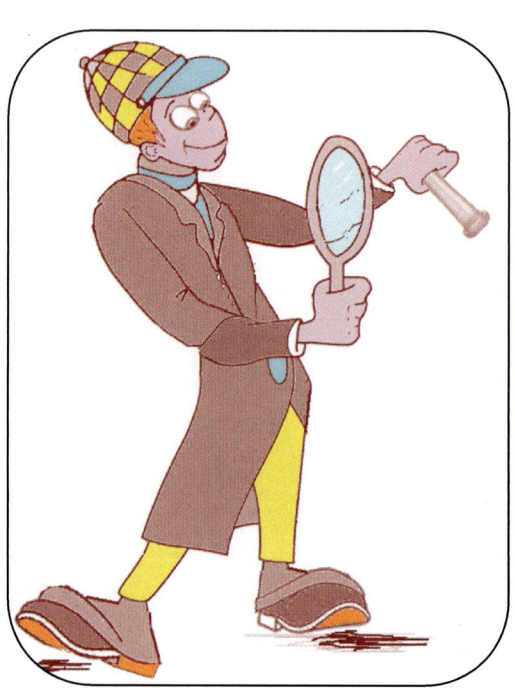

# PART 2 - COMPLEMENTARY COURSE

## Introduction

**In part 1**, we made a kind of ready-to-use (Quick Learning). That is, it required little knowledge. In this sequel, we will specify the lymphatic system and add some complementary movements.

## Veno-lymphatic drainage

### POSITION OF LYMPHATIC NODES

The treatment of facial drainage by cupping resumes in its main principles those of manual drainage. We start at the bottom to "empty" the lower lymphatic nodes, and then we go back gradually on each floor of the face. The upper part of the body and the face are interdependent by the connection of several lymphatic chains. These chains join the levels of lymphatic nodes (these are kind of crossroads). It is useful to represent them.

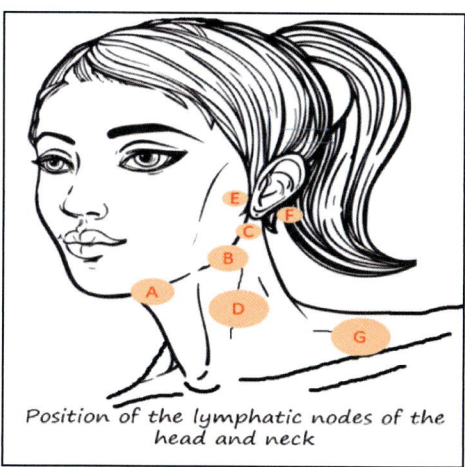

Position of the lymphatic nodes of the head and neck

A – Submentalis <u>n</u>odes (= **n.**). B – Sub mandibularis n. C - Sub parotid n.
D – Superior cervical n. E – Pre-auricular n. F – Retro-auricular n. G – Supraclavicular n.

# LYMPHATIC AND VENOUS DRAINAGE

The lymphatic and venous networks are very close with comparable paths. During facial cupping, there is therefore a venous drainage that is very conducive to the health of the face and its rejuvenation. It is a "valve" system that invites you to massage in one direction and go towards the direction of the heart. But at the level of the head, the system has no valves, which promotes drainage down (towards the heart). This also has a consequence of the numerous anastomoses of the deep venous network (inside the head) which can become engorged during a venous return in the opposite direction.

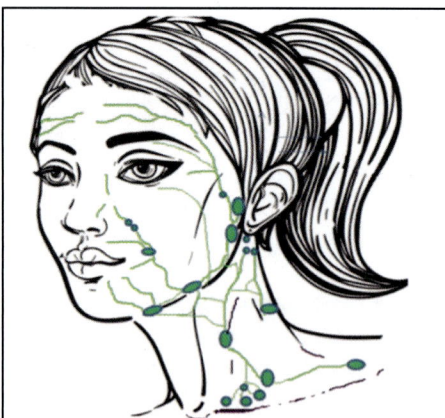

Position of the lymphatic chains and nodes of the head and neck

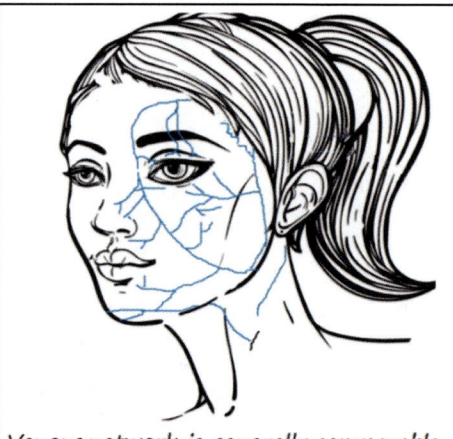

Venous network is generally comparable to the lymphatic network.

# With or without valves?

*...An important distinction...*

## GENERAL PRESENTATION OF THE LYMPHATIC SYSTEM

The lymphatic system is a network of ducts collecting the lymph (that is to say the liquid present between the cells). It starts with the lymphatic capillaries that are just under the skin and finally empties into the venous circulatory system through "branches" located just before the heart (called the thoracic duct and right lymphatic duct). It participates in the defense inmune because it is constituted of ganglia loaded (lymph nodes) with defense cells. The ganglia also serve to filter the lymph.

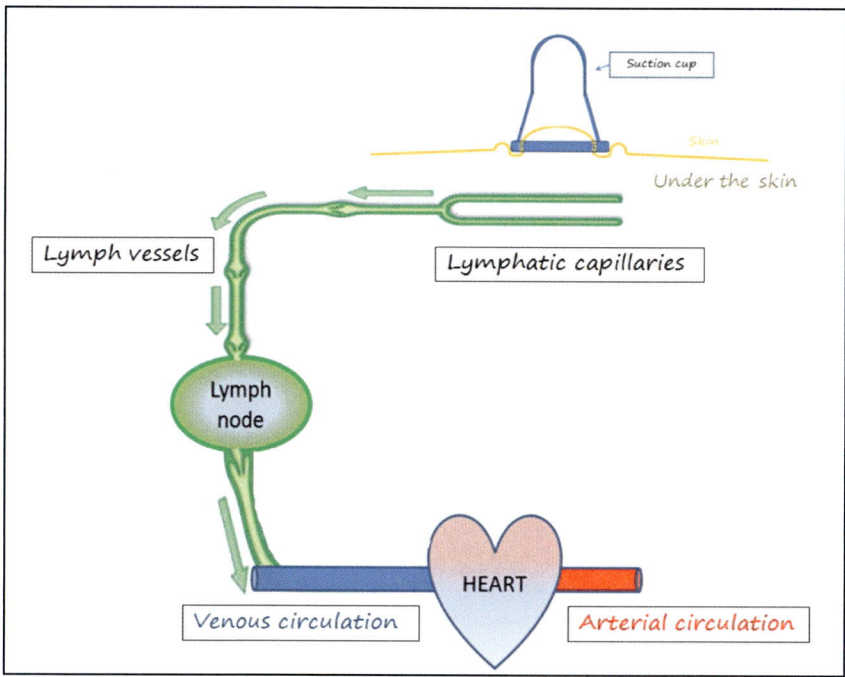

*Diagram of the lymphatic system.
Lymphatic capillaries are just under the skin...*

## LYMPHATIC CAPILLARIES WITHOUT VALVES

Lymphatic capillaries begin under the skin. In this area we also find venous and arterial capillaries. These are the smallest vessels in the lymphatic system. This situation under the skin of the capillaries will allow the use of suction cups for drainage, but also to release the fascias, the muscles. The other important feature of the capillaries: they have no valves, so that the lymph, depending on the circumstances, can flow in both directions. This is why the alternating movements of compressions and decompressions are interesting.

## LYMPHATIC VESSELS WITH VALVES

At a lower level under the skin, the lymphatic vessels have valves, that is to say it will circulate in one direction (they have different names depending on their size and anatomical situation such as pre-collector, collector ...). The presence of the valve "forces" veno-lymphatic drainage to be carried out in one direction, that is to say massage in the direction of venous return (to the heart, or the root of the limbs). Here, in this book, we talked about the Venus triangle (the root of the neck).

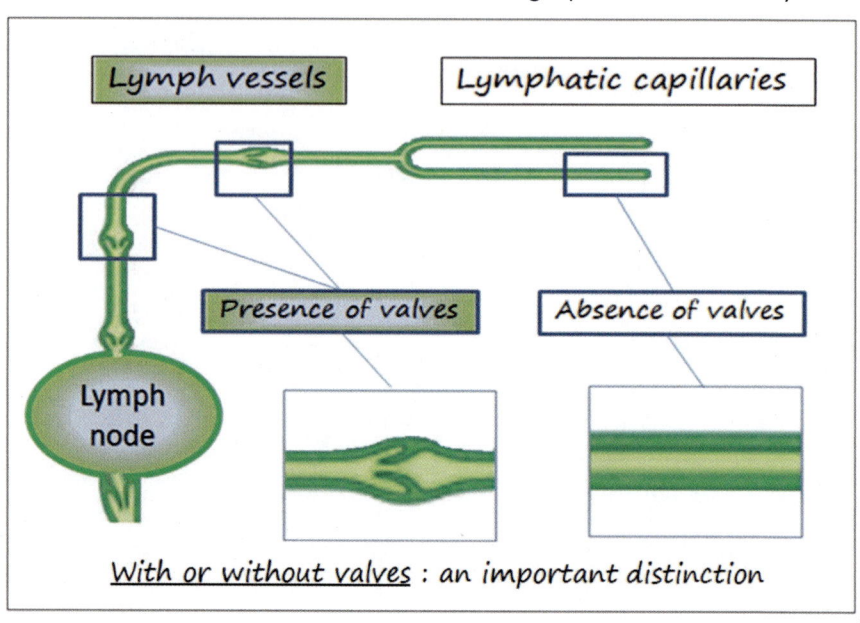

With or without valves : an important distinction

# SKIN AND LYMPHATIC CAPILLARIES

Lymphatics are a route of elimination and treatment of toxins. Participating in their drainage allows better health and have a less overloaded face and therefore fewer wrinkles. Despite the superficial aspect of the technique, its effect is profound. This is a unique technique that allows the opening of the lymphatic capillaries during the movements of the suction cup through the formation of a skin dome by negative pressure, that is to say during decompression.

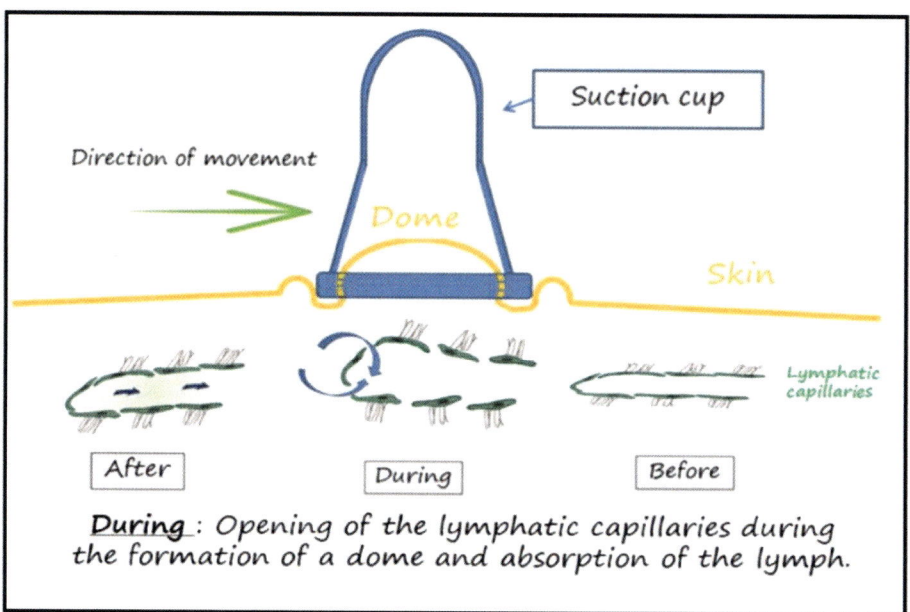

**During**: Opening of the lymphatic capillaries during the formation of a dome and absorption of the lymph.

Often when we talk about suction cup, we focus on the decompressive mechanism of vacuum suction. On the other hand, we often forget that the suction cup also has a double compressive effect by the application of these rims. There is even an alternation "compression - decompression - compression" during the movement, which sometimes "mimics" certain gestures of "compression and depression" during certain manual maneuvers without application of suction cups. This alternation obviously has an effect on the lymphatic vessels, but also on all the neighboring structures (blood vessels, collagen etc.).

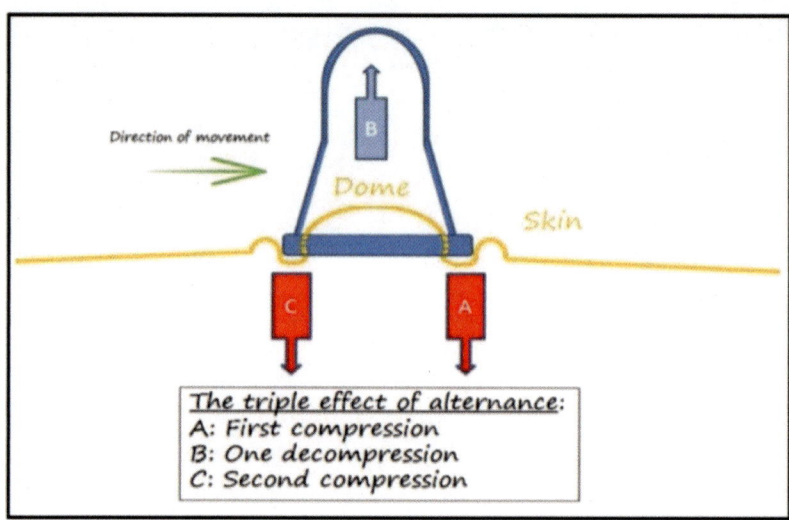

# ADDITIONAL MOVEMENTS FOR NECK AND FACE

## POSTERIOR REGION OF THE NECK

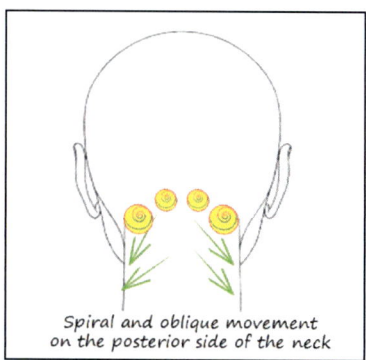

Spiral and oblique movement on the posterior side of the neck

During the facial cupping, if you have time, you can massage the back side of the neck. This is even advised in the books on lymphatic drainage. Of course, we do not work specifically on the face, but the head is an anatomical unit. In the same vein, it is useful to massage the region of the trapezium (not shown here).

## LONG JOURNEY MOVEMENT

This is one of the very specific movements of lymphatic drainage according to Emile Vodder. It starts from the root of the nose, through the "big ride" of the smile. The entire cheek and chin region are gradually treated to the sub-mentally and submandibular lymph nodes. Then we descend even further down to the triangle of Venus.

The particularity of the long journey: it is described as an essential movement draining the ganglia of the face and the cheek. It should be added that the large facial vein follows almost the same path! So we can say that it is veno-lymphatic drainage.

The advantage of the long journey: it is a movement that deeply drains the face from the lymphatic and venous point of view because the facial vein has branches (anastomoses) with veins coming from the depth of the face, the sinuses of the nose, eyes. We must also be careful to massage the lateral side of the neck because the facial vein connects to the internal jugular vein and also has an anastomosis with the external jugular vein!

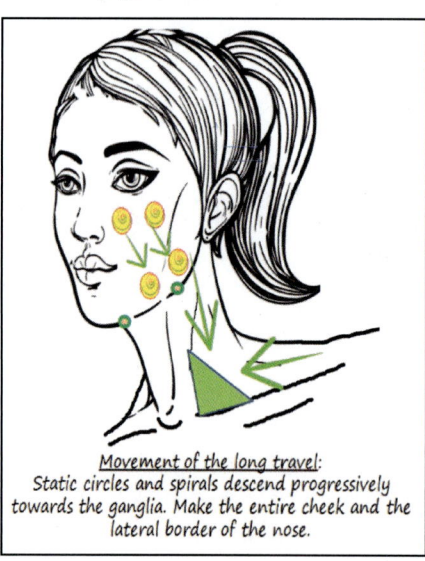

Movement of the long travel:
Static circles and spirals descend progressively towards the ganglia. Make the entire cheek and the lateral border of the nose.

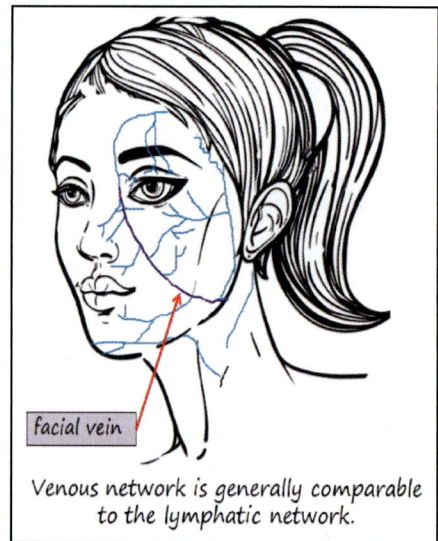

Venous network is generally comparable to the lymphatic network.

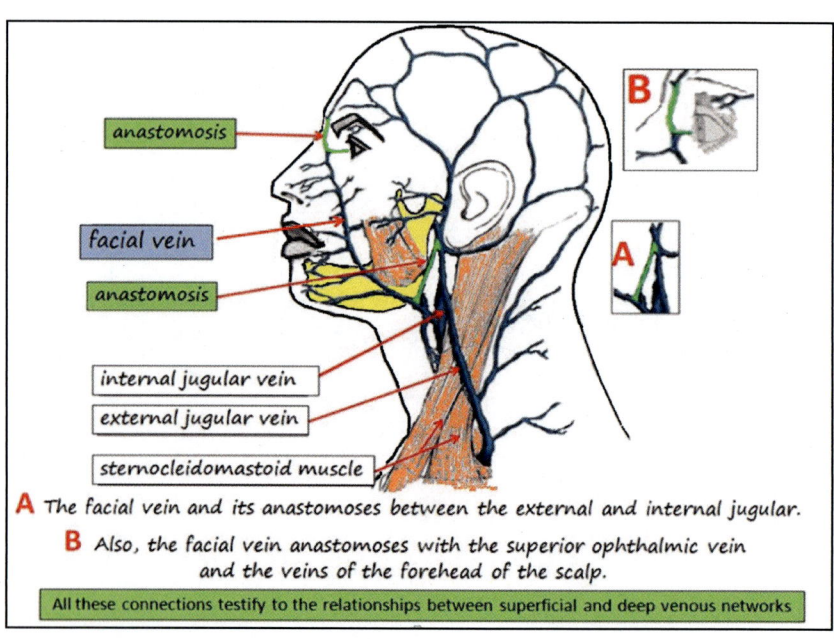

**A** The facial vein and its anastomoses between the external and internal jugular.

**B** Also, the facial vein anastomoses with the superior ophthalmic vein and the veins of the forehead of the scalp.

All these connections testify to the relationships between superficial and deep venous networks

# ADDITIONAL MOVEMENTS FOR EYES AREA

After making the movement of the long travel, *i.e.* drainage below the eyes, cheek and chin. You can do the drainage of the upper eyelids and eyes. It is an area overloaded with edema. For this, use a small silicone suction cup adapted to the thin skin of the eyelids.

## DRAINAGE DIRECTION IN THE EYELID AREA

The drainage of the eyelids is in two directions. The medial part (1/3 internal) drains towards the jaw, that is to say towards the mandibular nodes (hence the interest of having made the movement of the long travel). And the other part drains to the ear, that is to say to the pre-auricular nodes. Whether with the fingers or with a silicone suction cup, be sure to do both directions for a good evacuation of lymph and fluid in the eyelids.

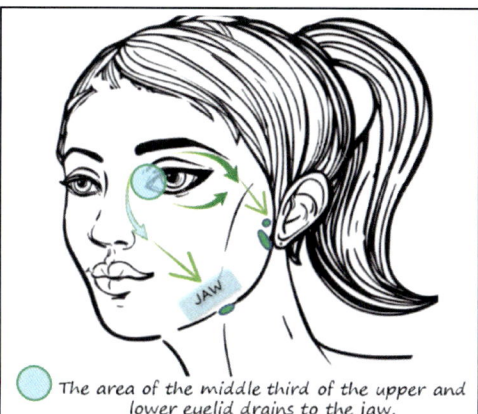

The area of the middle third of the upper and lower eyelid drains to the jaw.

We see in this diagram, the two directions for drainage. Also, Eyebrows drain to the ear.

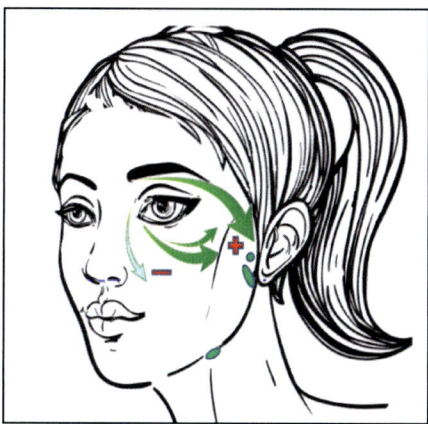

Recent studies have shown the preponderance (+) of the direction of eyelid drainage and eyebrows to the ear (the parotid). The entire eyelid may be involved in this direction. In practice cups, we will do both sides.

## OTHER OBSERVATIONS ON EYELID DRAINAGE

Note on the drainage of the upper eyelid: all the books do not agree, some exclude the upper eyelid of the drainage of the middle third. Similarly, some studies show drainage preferentially to the ear from the lymphatic system of the eyelids! However, it is important to keep in mind the two drainage directions. Everything remains to be discovered in terms of drainage of the eye and the eyelid!

A recent article (2015) gives us an indirect proof of the interest of a good drainage: Patients developed edema around the eye after using a C.P.A.P therapy. That is to say a mask that sends under pressure oxygen during sleep of the patient. The mask compresses the area of the face allowing drainage of the eyelid.

## EYELID, A PARTICULAR CROSSROADS OF DRAINAGE

Everything remains to be discovered in terms of eyelid drainage. Indeed, the lymphatic vessels of the eyelids form:

- A deep system that receives tarsus and conjunctiva from the eye.
- A superficial system that receives lymph from the orbicularis muscle and skin.

These two systems will then drain to the lymphatics of the face (to the ear first). But the lymphatics of the conjunctiva can collect liquid from inside the eye! (that is, the vitreous body).So, under certain conditions, they are the relay of evacuation of the lymph, if the eye cannot drain with the deeper lymphatics.

Facial cupping or manual drainage therefore has unsuspected deep effects other than reducing puffiness! These can be a reflection of an accumulation of waste from the depth of the face! Improvement of lymphatic and venous drainage pathways would provide new care paths for ophthalmologists. Indeed, the veno-lymphatic stasis of the orbit produces many problems.

# PUFFINESS DRAINAGE

### UNDERSTANDING

The drainage of the region of the eyelid and the cheek is not done with the same lymphatic vessels according to the anatomists. This delimitation is physical, that is to say that the eyelid has a very localized low limit: it is separated from the cheek by the orbicularis retaining ligament (ORL). It is a ligament that allows the separation of drainage. This ligament is on the rim of the orbit and the eyelid stops at the rim of the orbit! And many dark circles stop at the rim of the orbit! This is to understand that many dark circles following the retention of liquid (lack of drainage) stop on this rim. The Orbicularis Retaining Ligament (ORL) is a bit like sewing at the bottom of a pocket. On this circular ligament hangs a circular muscle, it is the "orbicularis muscle of the eyelids." It also helps to support all the soft structures present below the eye (muscle, fat, tarsus). What a champion this ligament!

The practical consequences of these remarks will be seen in the next section "practical remarks on movements". Now, it is useful to detail the surface anatomy and the relation of lymphatic drainage areas.

### SURFACE ANATOMY AND DRAINAGE

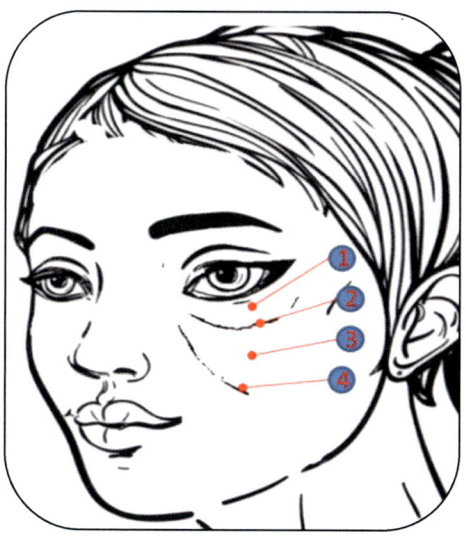

① Prolapsed orbital fat           ③ Malar bag
② Palpebro-malar groove (O.R.L)   ④ Midface groove (zygomatic cutaneous ligament)

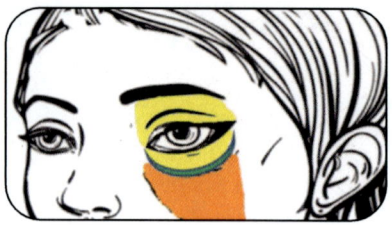
The lymphatic drainage areas are separated by the orbicularis retaining ligament (in green).

Lower portion of the orbicularis muscle separated by the ligament.

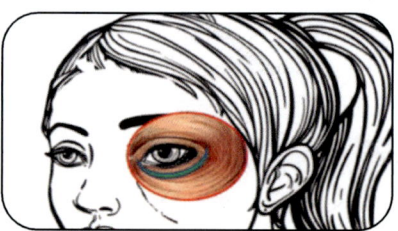

Diagram comments:

Dark circles and their limitations by the reticular ligament orbicularis (Green arched area). This ligament divides the two portions of the orbicularis muscle but also separates two drainage zones (in yellow and orange).

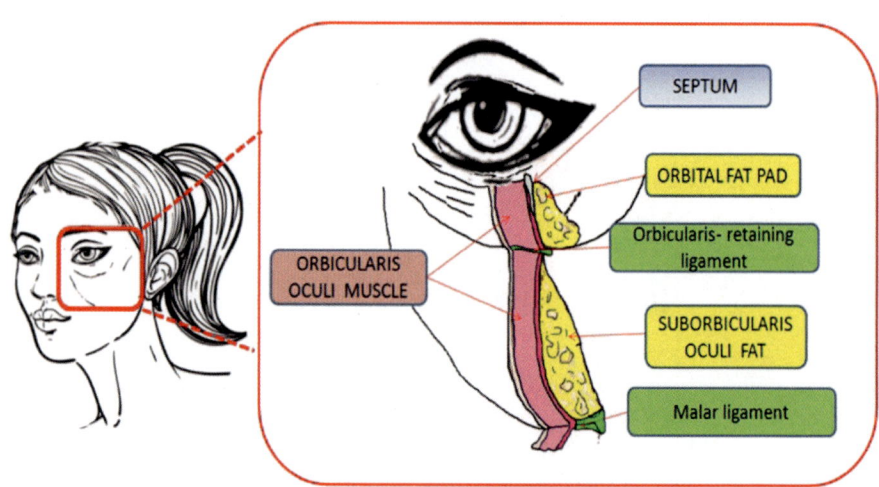

Details of the anatomy of delineation between eyelid and cheek.

Diagram comments:

We also note the presence of physiological fat packs. With age, inadequate nutrition, loosening of ligaments and tension of the skin or a vascular problem of veno-lymphatic drainage, these packets can increase in volume and aging the face with wrinkles.

Suckers can have general or localized effects on all these structures:

- Drainage effect and therefore decrease the fluid volume of the eyelids, respecting the evacuation routes.
- Cleaning effect because the eyelid is a drainage junction, it is a way of passage.
- Work wrinkles by lifting the skin tissue below the wrinkle (plumping effect).
- And if you are not afraid to create a little redness on the skin (effect of hyperemia): increase of the local vascularization with supply of nutrients for the structures concerned.

When we know the anatomical structures and the multiple effects of the suction cups, these small silicone objects are a real cosmetic surgery scalpel… It's up to you to try! And it is not forbidden to use the hands … It's up to you according to your feeling and experience.

## ADDITIONAL MOVEMENTS FOR SUBMANDIBULAR AREA

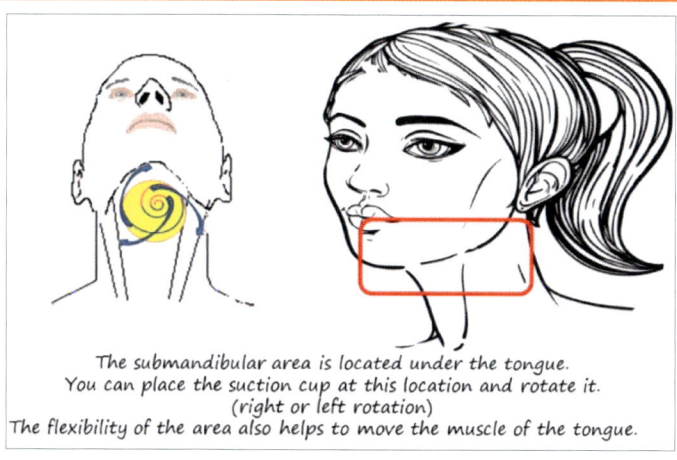

The submandibular area is located under the tongue.
You can place the suction cup at this location and rotate it.
(right or left rotation)
The flexibility of the area also helps to move the muscle of the tongue.

Under the jaw, the zone is flexible. You can place the suction cup for 30 seconds to a minute (fixed suction cup). This will attract toxins. Then move the sucker to the area of the star, that is to say the area of the parotid (mobile suction cup). It is a movement that can act deeply. Indeed, you mobilize the muscles of the oral floor (including the tongue). This will also reduce muscle tension.

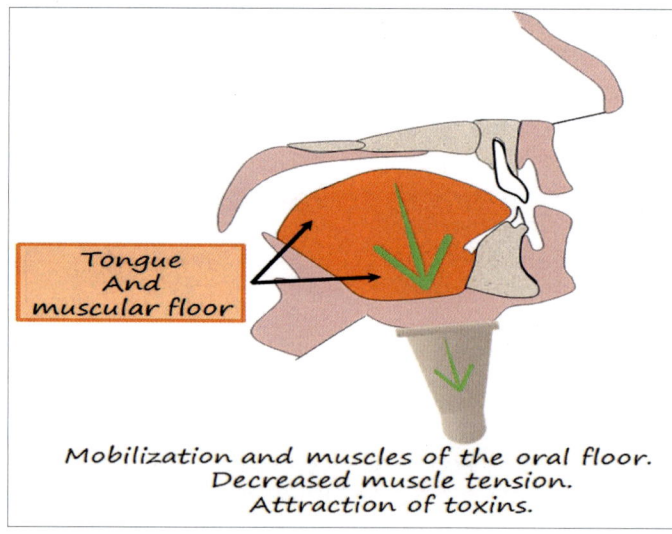

Mobilization and muscles of the oral floor.
Decreased muscle tension.
Attraction of toxins.

# REMARKS FOR ADDITIONAL MOVEMENTS

A – Drain in both directions of the eye:

According to recent studies, lymphatic drainage is mainly in the direction of the ear and the venous drainage goes to the root of the nose to join the facial vein. The two networks are intimately intertwined from a physiological point of view. As we have seen in paragraph of the long journey, the facial vein also passes over the inner corner of the eye and receives an anastomosis of an upper ophthalmic vein (hence from the depths of the orbit) and another from the forehead. Draining this area is also draining the eye from the venous point of view and not just the eyelids.

B – Locate the massage in the area of the eyelid, because the eyelid and the cheek are anatomical areas distinct from the point of view of lymphatic drainage. Make movements matching the curvature of the eyelids to the corners of the eye.

C – We can make **very soft glides** with small adapted suction cups, because this skin is one of the finest of the body! Some brief poses movements are possible (short pumping movement). Finally, the fingers are also ideal on the eyelids (even if in this book speaks of suction cups!).

D – Once you reach the corner of your eye, change to a bigger sucker to drain to the ear.

E – Application of fixed suction cups at parotid area (star area in our protocol of the first part of this book). If you have other plastic or glass suction cups, they can be useful for draining the drainage area of the ear. It's possible, if you are not afraid of some temporary red marks. Similarly, if you have a sufficient diameter of silicone suction cup, you can apply it to increase circulation. However, with silicone or plastic suction cups, you can adapt the pressure. Be careful, for this last point, if you do not want red marks; place the fixed suction cup at maximum for 2 minutes. But it also depends on your skin because some people blush more easily than others. Then, you can massage the area with your hands to disperse the fluids accumulated under the skin elevation.

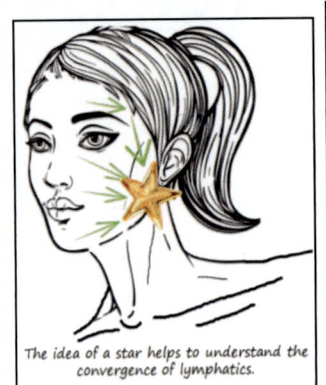

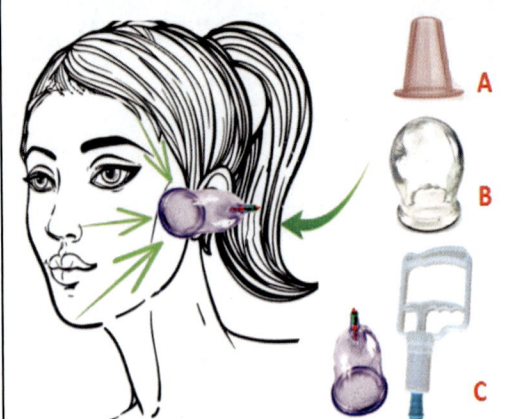

The idea of a star helps to understand the convergence of lymphatics.

Application of fixed suction cups on the area of the parotid (ear) to improve drainage of facial cupping.
Silicone (A), glass (B) or plastic (C) suction cups are possible.

# NERVOUS STIMULATION OF THE FACE

The lymphatic drainage of the face, as we saw above, provides venous drainage. Indeed, venous structures often follow the path of the lymphatic network. The superficial contact of the skin and the mobilization of the muscles, the suction cups also stimulate the nerves of the face and the neck.

In anatomical terms, the names of the nerves involved are: the facial nerve (number VII) and the trigeminal nerve (number V). Although they are distinct, these nerves have a synergistic action (in pain, touch and expression of emotions).

Lymphatic drainage is venous, but also, is nervous stimulation! Interestingly, these nerves that have branches in area are connected with brainstem structures!

The trigeminal nerve is the nerve of the pain of the head, neck and face! Most surprisingly, it is also connected (anastomosis) with nerves of the neck (vertebra C2 and C3). For this reason, you can have facial pains, while their origins come from the neck.

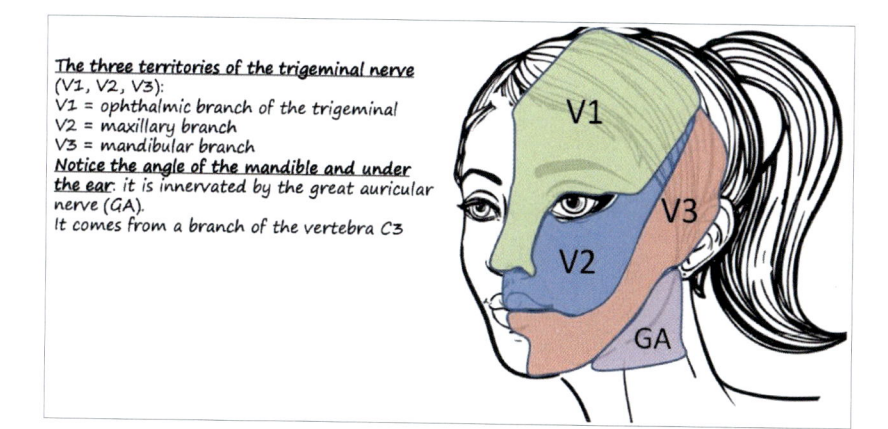

**The three territories of the trigeminal nerve** (V1, V2, V3):
V1 = ophthalmic branch of the trigeminal
V2 = maxillary branch
V3 = mandibular branch
**Notice the angle of the mandible and under the ear**: it is innervated by the great auricular nerve (GA).
It comes from a branch of the vertebra C3

# NERVOUS STIMULATION BETWEEN FACE AND BACK/NECK

For reasons of connection with face and cervical nerves, it is highly desirable, if you have time, to massage the neck area (with your hands or cupping). This will allow more relaxation of the face.

You can do the whole area of the neck, including the trapezius muscle with a bigger sucker. Many nerve connections exist between the back and the head, as we saw above. Even, if you do not know the anatomy of the muscles, feel the big muscular masses and follow their path.

This little book is an introduction to facial lymphatic massage. It aims to accompany the trainer and the student during an internship. That being said, we can illustrate an example of connection between the nerves of the face and the neck. We will do it with splenius muscle.

Indeed, the existence of nerve or muscle tension does not help natural lymphatic drainage. This is argued:
- Lymphatics are innervated and some types have a muscle wall.
- The lymphatic capillaries, located just under the skin, have anchoring filaments. These anchoring filaments strongly adhere to collagen and elastin of the skin.

## EXAMPLE OF SPLENIUS MUSCLES

Tensions, pains in the area of the gaze or on the top of the head can come from the neck. These pains cause tension, poor circulation of the face and lymph. A typical known example of trigger point manuals is the case of splenius muscles. In the plural, because splenius is composed of two muscles: the splenius of the head (= splenius capitis) and the splenius of the neck (= splenius cervicis).

They are important for the extension, rotation or lateral inclination of the neck and head. They are located under the trapezium.
- The splenius of the head can give pain to the top of the head.
- The splenius of the neck can give pain around the eye, in the area of the eyes.

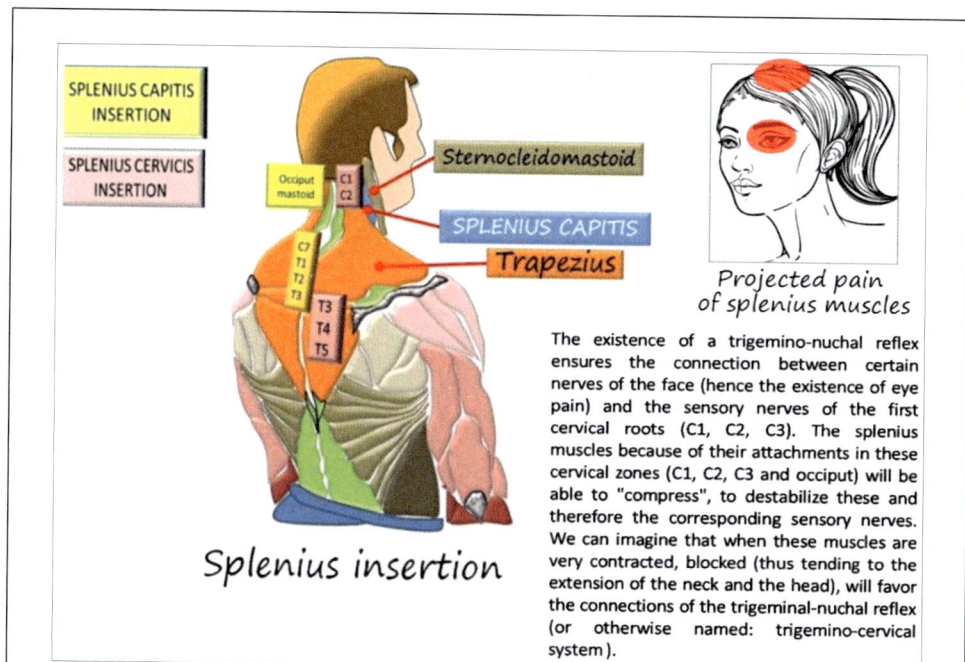

**SPLENIUS CAPITIS INSERTION**

**SPLENIUS CERVICIS INSERTION**

Sternocleidomastoid
SPLENIUS CAPITIS
Trapezius

Splenius insertion

*Projected pain of splenius muscles*

The existence of a trigemino-nuchal reflex ensures the connection between certain nerves of the face (hence the existence of eye pain) and the sensory nerves of the first cervical roots (C1, C2, C3). The splenius muscles because of their attachments in these cervical zones (C1, C2, C3 and occiput) will be able to "compress", to destabilize these and therefore the corresponding sensory nerves. We can imagine that when these muscles are very contracted, blocked (thus tending to the extension of the neck and the head), will favor the connections of the trigeminal-nuchal reflex (or otherwise named: trigemino-cervical system).

## MOBILE SUCTION STEP

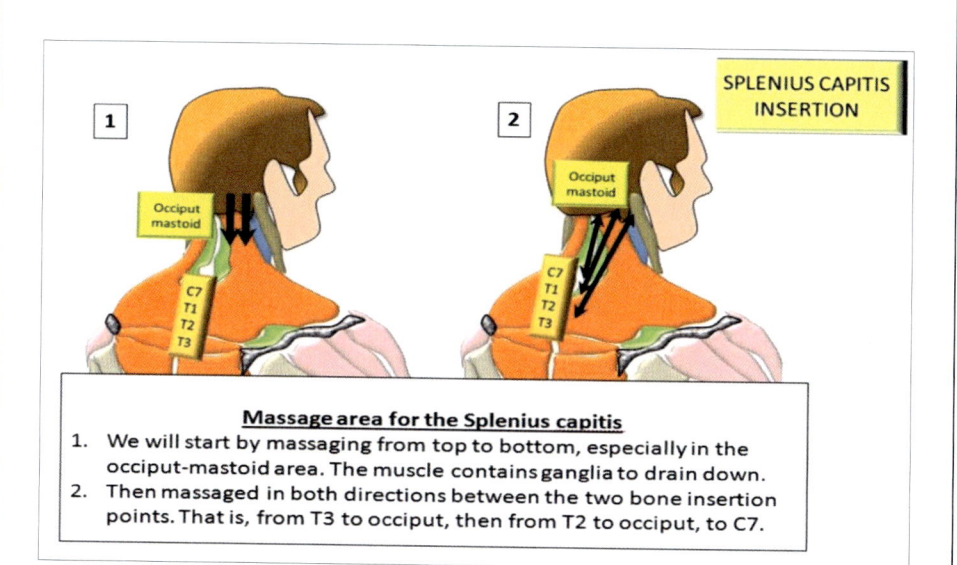

**SPLENIUS CAPITIS INSERTION**

### Massage area for the Splenius capitis

1. We will start by massaging from top to bottom, especially in the occiput-mastoid area. The muscle contains ganglia to drain down.
2. Then massaged in both directions between the two bone insertion points. That is, from T3 to occiput, then from T2 to occiput, to C7.

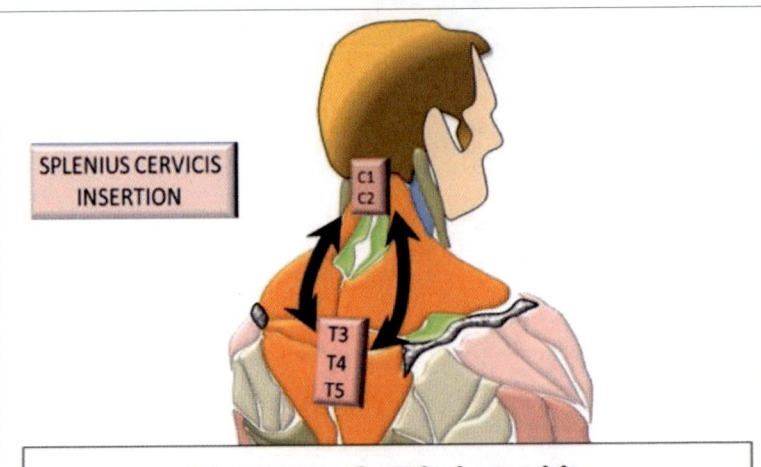

**SPLENIUS CERVICIS INSERTION**

**Massage area for Splenius cervicis**

It will be necessary to make "arcs of circle" going from T5 to C1, in order to follow anatomically the muscular bundles.

**FIXED SUCTION STEP**

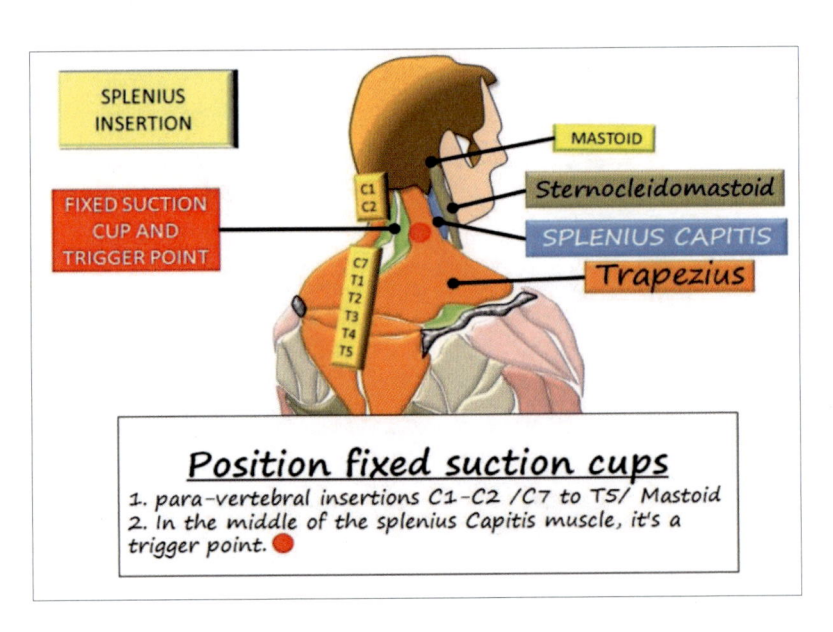

**SPLENIUS INSERTION**

**FIXED SUCTION CUP AND TRIGGER POINT**

MASTOID
Sternocleidomastoid
SPLENIUS CAPITIS
Trapezius

## Position fixed suction cups

1. para-vertebral insertions C1-C2 /C7 to T5/ Mastoid
2. In the middle of the splenius Capitis muscle, it's a trigger point. 🔴

**NOTES**

For more information on neuro-facial cupping. We have just published a new book, English and French version (January 2020).

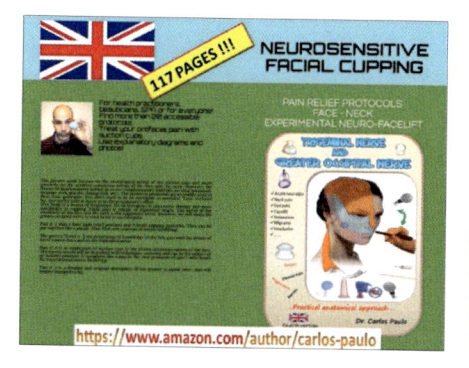

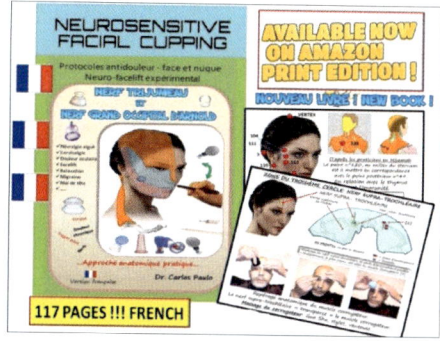

# Integrative Facial Cupping Part 3

## Cosmetic applications
## Face-lifting

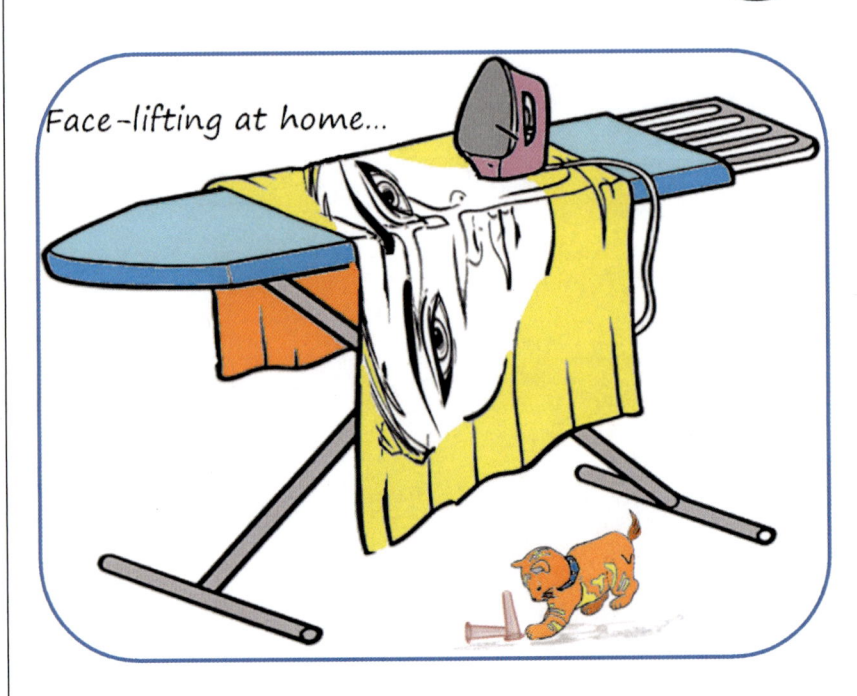

Face-lifting at home...

# PART 3 - FACE-LIFTING AND COMESTIC APPLICATIONS

## INTRODUCTION

In Part 2, we made a more precise study of lymphatic drainage. It is already a cosmetic application, because the suction cups are able to act on several systems at once. The lymphatic system allowed us a precise angle of view to work. In this part 3, we will of course focus on the cosmetic aspect that is not incompatible with lymphatic drainage. And no doubt, this is a highly anticipated chapter by the feminine genre interested in cupping facial and face-lifting.

## FACE-LIFTING PROTOCOLS

The different face-lifting protocols can be applied after drainage because the skin has been thoroughly cleansed, or separately during another session, so as not to stimulate the skin too much (if it has already reddened).

### DIFFERENCE BETWEEN LYMPHATIC DRAINAGE AND FACE-LIFTING

First, it's complementary. We will act here on the fast-circulatory system or on collagen. The hyperemic effect (specific to the suction cups) will be sought much more than in the lymphatic drainage.

Secondly, it is a more specific work for a clearer complexion of the face and wrinkles. Fixed suction cups will be added for a few minutes to bring "nourishing blood" to the face to revitalize it (fast-paced circulatory system). There is therefore a desired vascular effect more specifically than in drainage (although it may already be very present, when applying the Venus-Star protocol). Fixed plastic suction cups will be used, if you find that the vacuum is not strong enough with the silicone suction cups. The fixity of the suction cups must not exceed 3 minutes.

Thirdly, we will work in the "anti-wrinkle" direction, more specific movements towards the top of the face. A bit like the plastic surgeon stretching the skin upwards.

The lymphatic system is a system that goes down, and so sometimes the movement of the suction cups tends to go down. Which sometimes seems to go in the direction of a falling face. It is not, because it is a global and once completed drainage, it is possible to point the suction cups "upwards".

Also remember, that the lymphatic capillaries do not have valves, they can absorb the lymph coming from several directions under the skin of surface.

## HOW LONG TO TRY TO BE LESS RIDED?

The protocol will be carried out over several weeks (see 10 weeks with a rhythm of 2 to 3 times a week) with an effect from the first sessions. A clear effect will be visible around the sixth session for most people. Remember, repair processes in the body often take 6 weeks. When we do stretching, sport, it takes easily 6 weeks to adapt corporally. Note however, that it is not forbidden to make a light version of the protocols on a daily basis. To you to see and according to your experience.

## GRADUAL INTENSITY OF ASPIRATION

*...Progressively, increase the intensity of suction...*

In a cosmetic goal, practice the suckers very gradually. It involves gradually increasing the suction force to avoid red marks on the face. No strong suction immediately.

# CHEEK PROTOCOL

## INTRODUCTION

We call it so, because it will fight against the lines of tension of the face taking as a reference the zygomaxillary point and the pose of suction cups in this region. The movement will be upward across all anatomical parts without any real distinction as well as wrinkles. It goes in the opposite direction of a wrinkled face, it's a bit instinctive as a protocol. It is done in 2 steps that can be done independently. This protocol can be performed every day with 15 to 20 cup movements (one direction) for each treated area. It is a global massage of the face, because it is seen as a functional unit of which all the fibers must move upwards (in the direction of the smile).

## CHRONOLOGY

### First step: The upward orientation

The general direction of the suction cup is carried out thanks to a line having as points of intersection the central line and a second point well-known to plastic surgeons, the zygomaxillary point. The idea is to orient the structures of the face up, fighting against a "falling" face. The movement will be unidirectional; there will be no going back and forth to print "memory shape" to the skin. This protocol can be performed daily with 15 to 20 movements for each treated area. You can do it centimeter by centimeter with a suction cup size adapted to the anatomical region. Start with the chin and then gradually go up the central line.

### Second step: Fixed cups

Installation of a fixed suction cup on the cheek. In one sentence, it is to fight against the depressions of the cheek and eyelid interface caused by aging. This is a pose of suction cups on the cheek, in a short time of 2 to 3 minutes to bring blood to the face and have a plumping and anti-atrophic effect. You will see during this suction also that the lower part of the face will go up.

## SECOND STEP: VARIANT

Another variant is to make brief poses of a few seconds over the entire area of the middle face. Personally, we like to do it with manual pump plastic suction cups. You need to make a single gentle suction pressure with brief poses. Plastic suction cups will also draw more blood into the face. If you do not have this type of pumps, you can do it with silicone suction cups.

**CAUTION FOR THE SECOND STEP**: During this pose, avoid the area of the eyelids so that they are not attracted by suction cups. Personally, we like to do it with plastic suction cups with manual pumps. Check if you have too strong red marks. If you have any doubt about it, put the sucker for 30 seconds to 1 minute, and then do the verification. If you blush too much with marks, you can stop if you wish.

### ILLUSTRATION

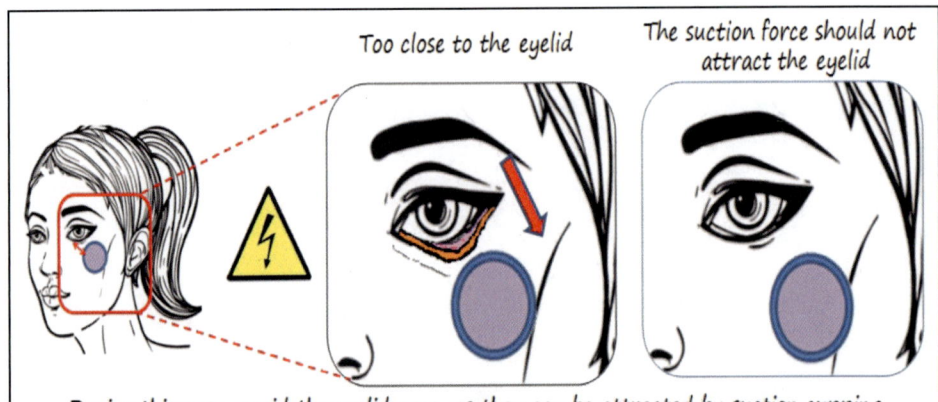

Too close to the eyelid

The suction force should not attract the eyelid

During this pose, avoid the eyelid area, as they can be attracted by suction cupping. Do not get close to avoid deforming the septum (cartilaginous structure of the eyelid).

## First step

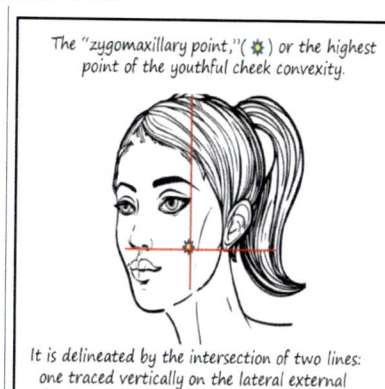

The "zygomaxillary point," (✻) or the highest point of the youthful cheek convexity.

It is delineated by the intersection of two lines: one traced vertically on the lateral external orbital rim, and another horizontally from the upper lateral cartilage of the nose to the tragus.

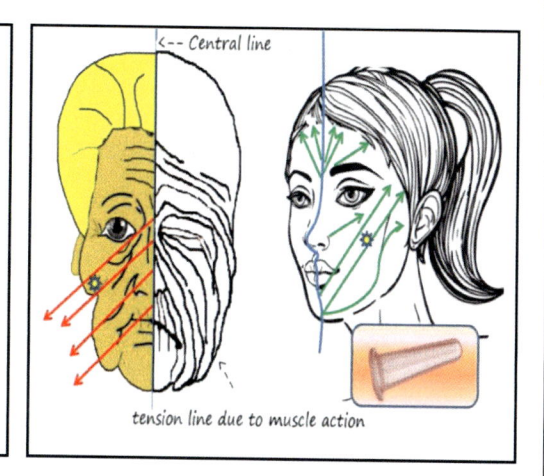

<-- Central line

tension line due to muscle action

## Second step

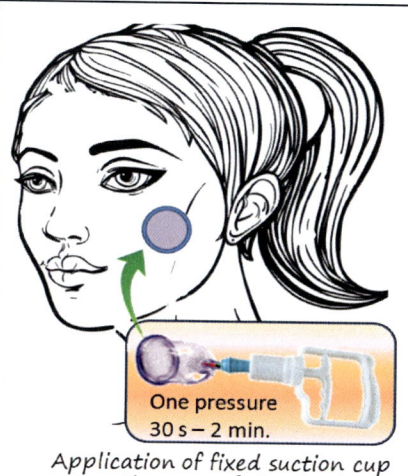

One pressure
30 s – 2 min.

Application of fixed suction cup on the area of the cheek.
<u>Time</u>: Less than 2 minutes, or depending on your experience (30 seconds, 1 minute).

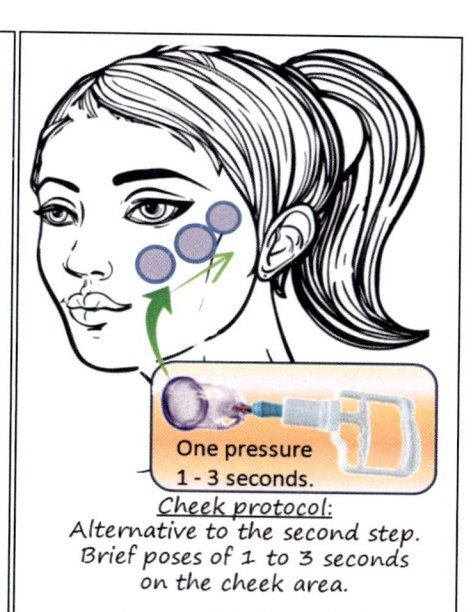

One pressure
1 - 3 seconds.

<u>Cheek protocol:</u>
Alternative to the second step. Brief poses of 1 to 3 seconds on the cheek area.

# REASONING

## FIRST STEP

### Stretching property

We therefore take advantage of the natural property of elongation of the skin by sucking the suction cups, by raising the skin and using a general direction of the suction cups to the top of the face. Imagine a surgeon pulling your skin from the temples!

### The change of shape of the face

Cosmetic surgeons know it well, the face changes over time. Certain areas are characteristic and form a pivot in this change, such as the descent of the zygomaxillary point, which defines a convex area of the cheek giving a pulpy, youthful aspect to the face. That's why we talk about it in this protocol. This descent of the skin indicates a "loosening" of the underlying soft structures then involving the wrinkles (we talked about it briefly in Part 2, during the precise anatomical delineation of the eyelid). Wrinkles and lines of tension are also "printed" because of the daily action of the muscles of the face. This relaxation gives a face appearance falling and wrinkled.

## SECOND STEP

### Against the loss volume

It is the natural history of the aging of the cheek region that gives a falling and less pulpy appearance. The application of fixed suction cup aims to feed the area of the cheek and plump. Indeed, this area is the site of several grooves (nasojugal and orbitomalar groove) whose digging effect is increased by a loss of tissue volume with the age and volume of fat present in the lower eyelid. .All this will form a "V" deformation of this part of the face that must be erased with the suction cups. Erase the "V", surgeons know it well, because they go as far as injecting belly fat into the periorbital zone and the cheek, during cosmetic surgery operations, according to the knowledge of this loss of volume!

As it is said in the precautions, it will be necessary to avoid the zone of the eyelid and the deformation of the cartilaginous septum (tarsus) by the suction of the sucker. Why? This one becomes more deformable with time. Sometimes, in some people, there is a pseudohernia (eyelid that falls with age) that adds to the aging effect of a face. The skin and the face have a memory of form and the objective of this protocol is not to make fall the eyelids! Please watch out for the extended skin area stretched by the suction cup so as not to move the tarsus down.

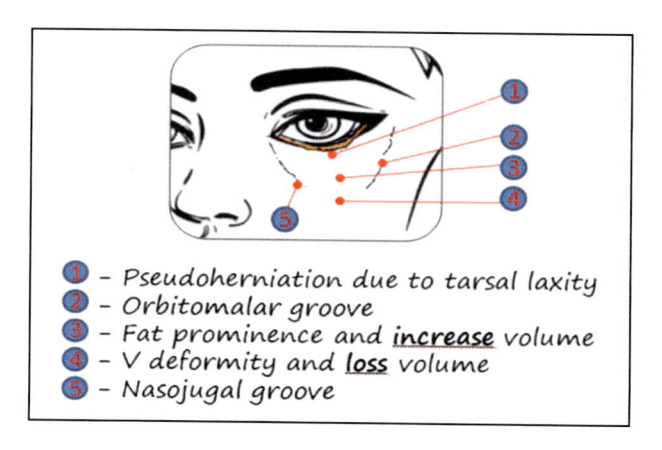

① - Pseudoherniation due to tarsal laxity
② - Orbitomalar groove
③ - Fat prominence and *increase* volume
④ - V deformity and *loss* volume
⑤ - Nasojugal groove

Effect aging and midface. These 5 points of anatomy are to be considered in the cheek protocol.

## CONCLUSION

In Part 2 of this book, we talked about the drainage of the eyelid. Indeed, the lower eyelid can be "inflated" by its fatty anatomical structures but also by the overload of the lymphatic network. We will try to reduce the volume with drainage. While in the protocol of the cheek, we will seek to plump the neighboring areas of the eyelid, especially for people with a "digging".

In all, whether using drainage or cheek protocol, the general aspect of the gaze will be worked with a harmonization of the volumes of the different zones, that is to say towards a general flattening of the hollows. A hollow can be filled by its groove (plumping effect) or can be reduced by decreasing the size of the next higher zones (drainage effect of the lymph). From a physiological point of view, it is better to start with the "Venus-Star" protocol, because once the lymph is gone (drained), the nourishing blood is brought in with the fixed suction cups. We admit that this order can be discussed according to your experience.

# Rejuvenation protocol

### INTRODUCTION

We will describe the program of Mr. Chirali Ilkay Zihni described in his book on cupping: the "facial rejuvenation". The goal is to put fixed suction cups on the face for 2 to 3 minutes and apply mobile suction cups. All systems participating in the youth of the face are activated as:

- Blood loaded with nutrients and oxygen.
- Activation of lymphatic drainage.
- Stimulation of elastin and collagen.

We note, therefore, that the *Venus-Star* protocol is complete with that of Mr. Chirali. He added notions of Chinese medicine that will be treated little in this book but whose author is constantly referring in his book (see references).

### CHRONOLOGY

The author proposes a treatment twice a week over 6 weeks with a visible effect at the end of the sixth session. It proposes a progression in the increase of the suction force of the suction cups. Chirali describe two Importants steps in its treatment (Mobile and fixed suction cups).

First step: Mobile

The mobile suction cups, themselves subdivided into two phases: the face and the eyes. Rubber or silicone suction cups are readily used.

The face: Starting at the top of the face, that is to say the middle of the forehead. Here is the order of succession: forehead, face, under the eyes, nose, lips, in front and then behind the ears to finish on the neckline. Make 5 to 7 long movements in one go all the reliefs of the face.

Eyes: Starting from the top of the face, that is to say the middle of the forehead and just above the eyebrows. Then follow the edge of the orbit by a circular motion joining the inner corner of the eye. Make 15 to 20 movements at each visit. Note: the passage through the outer corner of the eye goes through an acupuncture point called TAIYANG. If you do not know how to spot the TAIYANG, this should not prevent you from doing the global move.

## SECOND STEP: FIXE

Plastic suction cups with manual pump are readily available. He does not really specify a place, but we can notice in his book that he proposes to place 2 medium-sized fixed suction cups just below the temple and the lateral rim of the mouth.

These positions are good for two reasons:

    1 - There is a lateral stretching of the skin which allows to "lifter" the skin.

    2 - They are placed on the large venous and lymphatic drainage paths.

From a cosmetic point of view to avoid making strong red imprints, the plastic suction cups stay in place no more than three minutes. The time of fixity also depends on the patient and her skin; do not hesitate to remove them to test the redness after 30 seconds to a minute.

## ILLUSTRATION

This book does not deal with Chinese medicine. We put some precision on the points of acupuncture, because the author Chirali relies much on the Asian notions.

## First step: Mobile

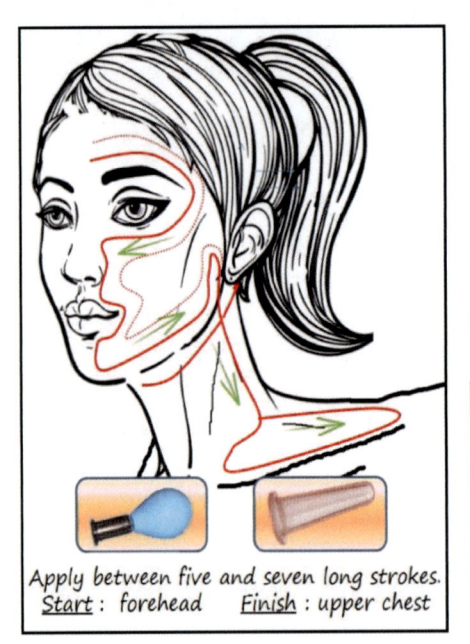

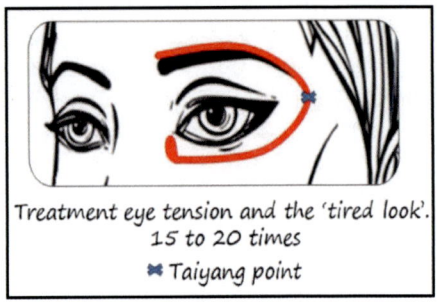

Treatment eye tension and the 'tired look'.
15 to 20 times
✹ Taiyang point

Point to improve eyesight and eye tension

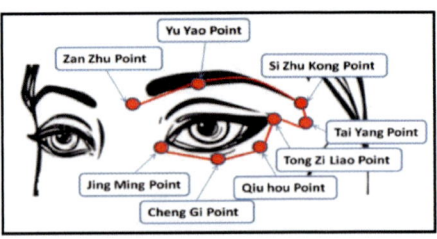

Yu Yao Point
Zan Zhu Point
Si Zhu Kong Point
Tai Yang Point
Tong Zi Liao Point
Jing Ming Point
Qiu hou Point
Cheng Gi Point

Apply between five and seven long strokes.
<u>Start</u> : forehead    <u>Finish</u> : upper chest

Step of the mobile suction cup in the facelift according to the book of Chirali. Face and eye protocol. The different points of acupuncture can be stimulated by the path of the silicon cup.

## Second step: Fixe

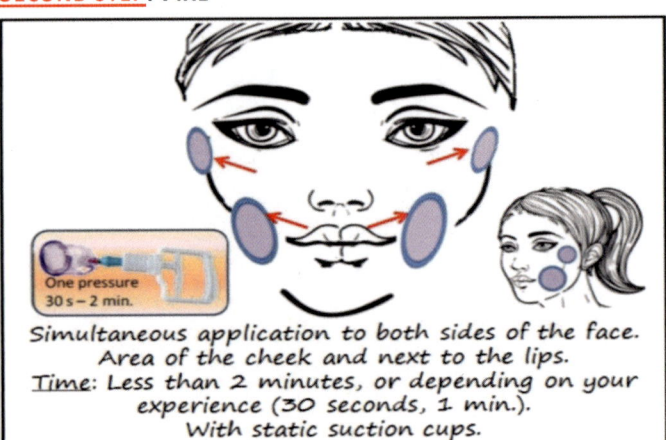

One pressure
30 s – 2 min.

Simultaneous application to both sides of the face.
Area of the cheek and next to the lips.
<u>Time</u>: Less than 2 minutes, or depending on your experience (30 seconds, 1 min.).
With static suction cups.

### The goal:

To bring oxygenated blood to the face. With the sessions, there will be a shine on the face with an effect of vitality and youth.

# THREE FORCES PROTOCOL

## INTRODUCTION

This protocol is inspired by the mechanical properties of the skin by applying 3 constraints: rotation, vertical tension up (suction - decompression) and vertical tension down (compression) by manual massage (hand or Gua Sha instrument). The goal is to stimulate the deep planes of the skin and the synthesis of collagen present under the skin. Rotations should not be constraining, please be gentle in the application of the protocol.

This protocol consists of three stages:

- Rotary,
- Smoothing wrinkles (vertical tension up),
- Longitudinal with compression (vertical tension down).

## CHRONOLOGY

<u>FIRST STEP</u>: ROTATION

**Application of a torsion force**. Rotational movements should be measured so as not to wrinkle the skin in the wrong direction. For this, start with a suction pressure (see maximum 2) with the plastic hand pump to test the skin. Rotations should be made outward (towards the ear) from the centerline. The pose will be soft with rotation of the suction cup. Browse all the face from bottom to top, much like in the "cheek protocol" but with the rotations. Avoid getting too close to the eyelids, because the skin becomes very thin to make rotations. Too close to the eyelids can cause pain and lowering them.

It will be necessary to adapt the suction pressure to the sensation of the patient. Plastic hand pumps will be preferred to hope to reach the deeper integuments. You can do this also with silicone suction cups. If you feel that the patient does not support rotations and stimulation, stop the protocol. And work in a softer way. Browse the face from the bottom up, the patient must have a deep working feeling at the end of the session.

### SECOND STEP: SMOOTHING

Applying a vertical force upwards (decompression). It is a very soft massage with silicone suction cups. For this step, we follow the path of the wrinkle with a back and forth movement (a little as if we use a flat-iron in a fold of clothes). It will act as a "plumping" and hyperemia effect thanks to its vertical upward suction force that will attenuate the hollow of the wrinkle. Do at least 3 movements back and forth.

### THIRD STEP: COMPRESSION

Additional step of manual massage *i.e.* Applying vertical force down (compression). Either with bare hands or with a GUA SHA type instrument. The GUA SHA instrument is well-known in Chinese medicine. If you do not have one, you can use a porcelain spoon and "smooth" the skin with it. Always in a gentle way, it will stimulate the skin down. There will also be a stretch of the skin. Movements will resume those of the "cheek protocol" or the "Venus-Star protocol".

## ILLUSTRATION

### FIRST STEP: ROTATION

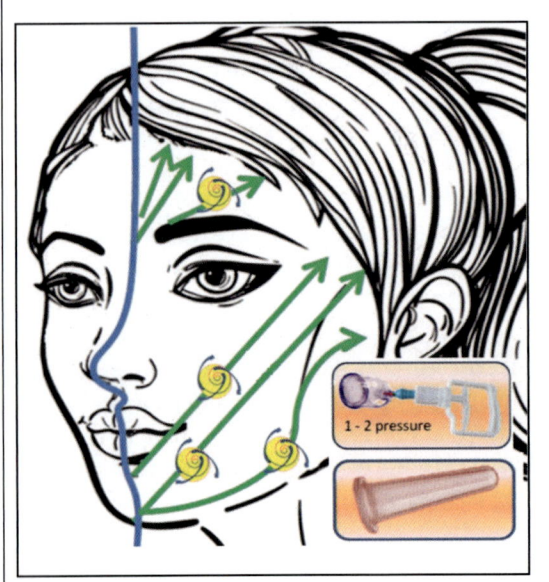

Rotations should be made outward (towards the ear) from the centerline. We must not force, it is just moving the deep plans without exaggeration of the rotation.

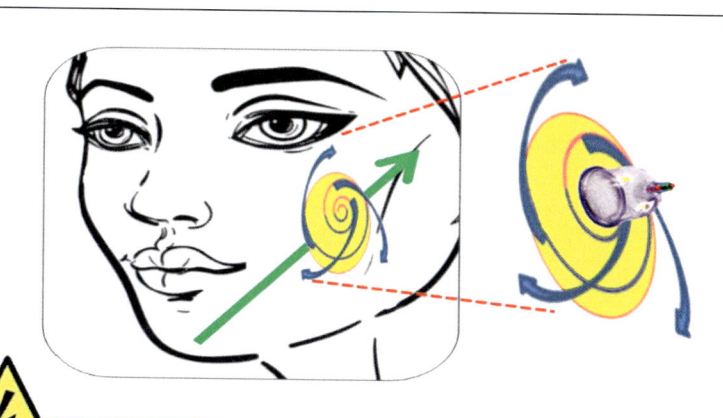

Rotations must be gentle.
This is not a test of mechanical resistance of the skin!
Adapt to the patient and her feeling.
It is not necessary to provide a strong redness.

## Second step: Smoothing

We will work in the direction of the length of the different wrinkles. Make at least 3 round trips on each wrinkle. You can start with the top of the face or the bottom.

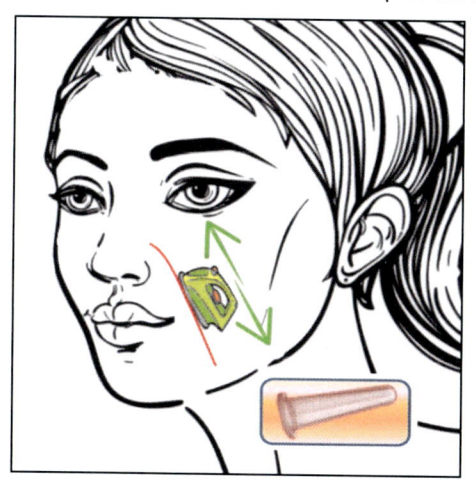

### THIRD STEP: COMPRESSION

For this third step, we refer you to the "Venus-Star Protocol" (Part 1) and the "Cheek Protocol" schemas (Part 3). Indeed, these are transposable for manual application or application by friction using an instrument.

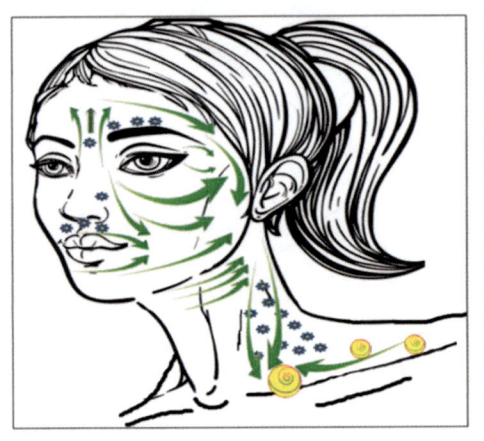

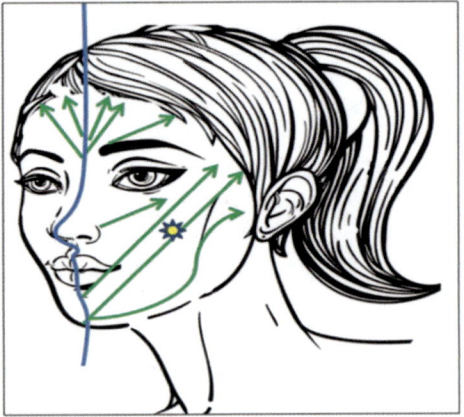

Venus-Star protocol (Lymphatic drainage)

Cheek protocol (facelifting)

## REASONNING

**FIRST STEP**

Gentle rotatory step

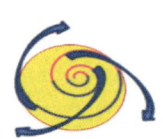

The rotary step is inspired by Jacquet-Leroy pinches for the treatment of scars and wrinkles. They are commonly used by the beautician with the hands. The pinches must be vigorous and fast to be able to "catch" the muscle and twist it. Jacquet's pinching is a deep stimulation of the skin and not its surface. Some women are fond of these. With cupping, we cannot do as fast as the hands, as do beauticians and it is not about "tearing" the skin. Care should be taken to make gentle rotations. The technique should not be painful, but feeling a "tug" of the skin is normal. Blood is brought to the skin to revitalize it by rotating the suction cup (imitating pinching). The dermis and the muscles of the face are also stimulated.

*In total, the application of forces can be summarized as:*

TORSION + <u>DE</u>COMPRESSION

## SECOND STEP

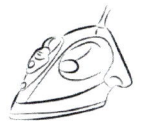

Smoothing wrinkles step

After having stimulated the skin with rotations, we work in the direction of the length of a specific wrinkle. Here too, we are inspired by the work on scars and certain movements well-known to beauticians for wrinkle removal work. This work of smoothing wrinkles will associate gladly with very gentle massage cupping all over the face. That is to say, we will rather use silicone suction cups after stimulating the skin rotationally.

*In total, the application of forces can be summarized as:*

LONGITUDINAL STRETCHING + **DE**COMPRESSION

## THIRD STEP

Soft compression step

The goal will not really be to recreate a hyperemia (a redness of the skin) as in the real Gua Sha, but to stimulate, to give compression information to the skin. This gentle compression will also open the lymphatic capillaries, for that you can resume the steps of the "cheek protocol" or the massage with the hand by taking again the protocol "Venus-Star" of the part 1.

*In total, the application of forces can be summarized as:*

LONGITUDINAL STRETCHING + COMPRESSION

# Integrative Facial Cupping
# Part 4

## Complementary methods

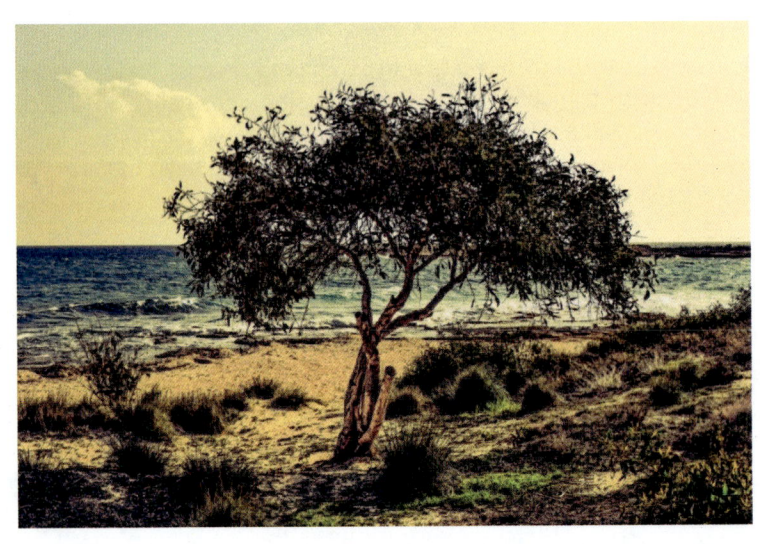

*The olive tree, a friend for the beauty of your face.*

# PART 4 - COMPLEMENTARY METHODS

## INTRODUCTION

**In Part 3**, we made a more precise study of face-lifting. It leads us to consider the face and the head as a functional anatomical unit. Indeed, the superficial structures of the face are in relation with the deep structures. This functional unit is itself made up of different functional units (a bit like Russian dolls). Thus, the anatomical unit of the cheek is in relation with the functional unit of the eye. And the eye is in relation with the brain...

**In this part 4**, we will use some complementary methods for facial drainage, good facial health. There will also be some additional tips and anatomical notions. We will quote two, well-known naturopaths:

- The nasal shower or Jala Neti practiced by the yogis for many centuries and taken over by Finnish otolaryngologists.
- The mouthwash oil, detoxifying and draining.

A third less known technique will also be mentioned:

- Massage Meibomian glands with a kind of small plastic "clip" that allows better drainage of the eyelid and better moistening of the eye.

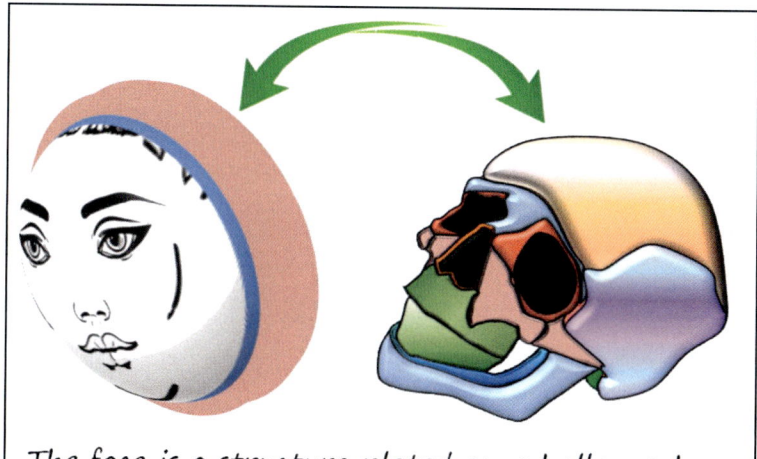

*The face is a structure plated on a hollow sphere that is called the head or skull.*

# WHICH OIL CAN I USE?

### THE VARIOUS OILS POSSIBLE

From this point of view, you can trust your beautician who certainly has her beauty secrets! However, it is usual to use jojoba oil or coconut oil. They are numerous and varied in parapharmacy. Some creams or oils are made with collagen or vitamin C. It's up to you to choose what you prefer. The important thing is that it can slide well with the sucker! As part of this book on facial cupping and the desire to have fewer wrinkles, we will advise you to use olive oil.

### WHY OLIVE OIL?

Because it is easily found, preferably biological and it is economical. It has an excellent tolerance to the skin and is composed of many nutrients. As a result, it is suitable for all types of skin. Many people traditionally use it for beauty and health care. It is also known as anti-wrinkle. It can also be a good makeup remover before using suction cups!

Interestingly, you can combine another substance with olive oil. Indeed, it promotes skin penetration of active substances such as essential oils or polyphenols such as quercetin according to recent studies. It has an excellent synergy with good natural products. You can even enrich your anti-wrinkle cream with a few drops of essential oils! Your turn to try! As part of this book, we can recommend the wonderful lemon drops after pressing or essential oil.

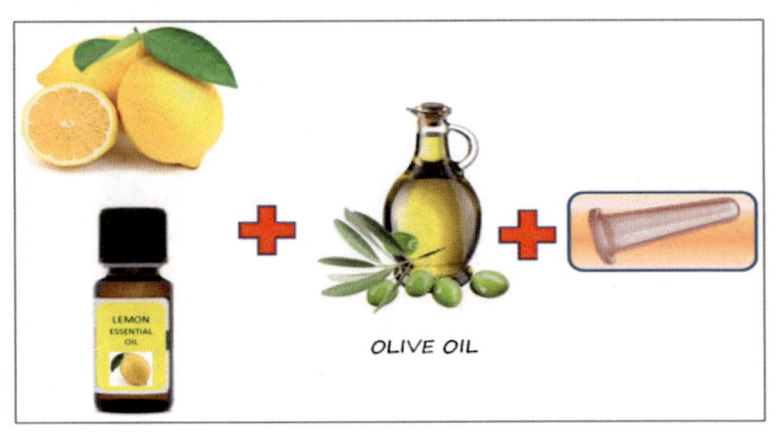

*A few drops of lemon and olive oil.*
*An option for facial cupping.*

# JALA NETI

## DESCRIPTION

By typing the word "Jala Neti" on the search engine "Google" or Youtube, you will easily find tutorials on the nasal shower. We urge you to do so as part of this book. We will briefly describe the technique and expose some reasoning on the benefits and the links with cupping facial.

### MATERIAL

- A small teapot or container that yogis call "Neti lota",
- Warm water (around 32 ° C),
- A teaspoon or tea of salt (sea) for 500 ml of water (1/2 liter).

### TECHNIQUE

- Put the beak in the nostril, and then tilt the head while raising the teapot or Lota.
- The water that enters through one nostril leaves through the other nostril. Pass at least 500 ml in each nostril.
- At the end of the technique, thoroughly dry the nasal cavities! They must be dry at the end of the technique. To do this, make 30 breaths or exhalations in each nostril to evacuate water and moisture.

It can be done daily in the morning, or more often in case of congestion or colds.

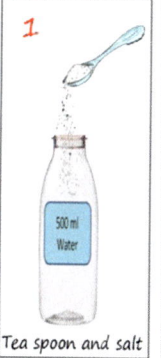

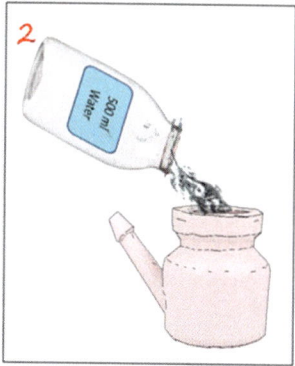

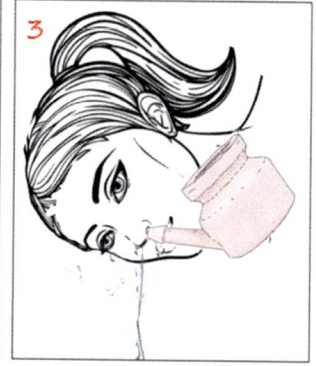

## REASONING

Jala Neti cleans the nasal cavity and relieves all nearby anatomical structures and their associated symptoms. Less nasal congestion allows the free passage of air, less allergy and dust. This will affect the health of the face, if it drains deeply, this will be seen on the surface. Indeed, we saw in part 2 that the deep veins are in relation to the superficial veins. This is also the case for the lymphatic network. In addition, having decongested nasal passages allows less congestion in the eyelids. Indeed, the lacrimal duct is a neighbour very close to the nasal cavity. A disturbance of this network will tend to swell the eyelids. Very often, allergic, smokers have overloads in the eyelids.

# OIL THERAPY IN THE MOUTH

### DESCRIPTION

It's a mouthwash with oil every morning to clean the mouth and drain toxins from the entire area of the face, throat and even the body. Indeed, the lining of the mouth is an "interface" of exchange. Ayurveda naturopaths are familiar with this method.

**MATERIAL**

- Sunflower or ajonjoli oil, first cold pressed.

**TECHNIQUE**

- Application in the morning, before breakfast.
- Take a tablespoon of oil without swallowing.
- Then slowly, move the oil in the various parts of the mouth.
- Make a good impregnation of the mouth with the oil for 3 to 4 minutes. Oil mixes with saliva and enzymes.

After several minutes, the appearance of the oil will change due to its load of toxins and the presence of cell debris of bacterial origin. It will be milky (white) or opaque. Repeat this application several times. The author Andreas Moritz in his book on cleaning on the liver advises to do it 3 times a day on an empty stomach (empty stomach) in case of illness. Then rinse your mouth with baking soda and wash your teeth.

### REASONING

The goal is to cleanse the body, eliminate toxins through the oil that will attract toxins and promote the relief of organs such as the liver and nearby structures such as the face and the lymphatic system. The face is an anatomical functional unit as we said before, anything that helps to alleviate the face in the deep structures will allow a new vitality of the same. The mouth is a gateway for the entry and exit of toxins that needs to be considered in the concept of integrative facial cupping.

# DRAINAGE GLAND OF MEBOMIAN

## DESCRIPTION

**MATERIAL**

- You need a device called: Eyepeace®.

**TECHNIQUE**

- Squeeze and release, 5 – 10 times on each eye.
- Make for 2 minutes twice a day and can be combined with hot compresses.

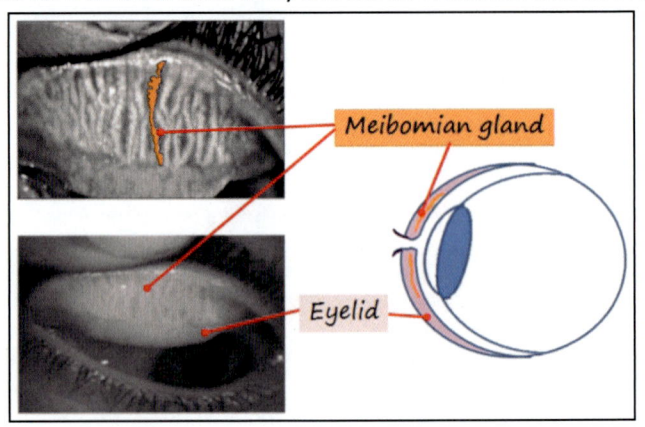

Meibography image taken with the Oculus ® Keratograph 5M (see references).

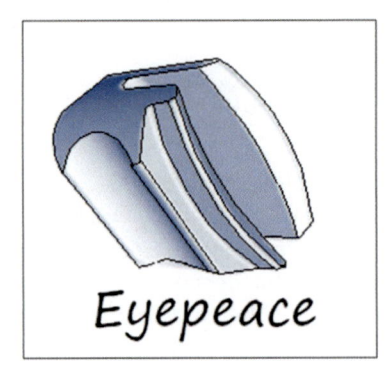

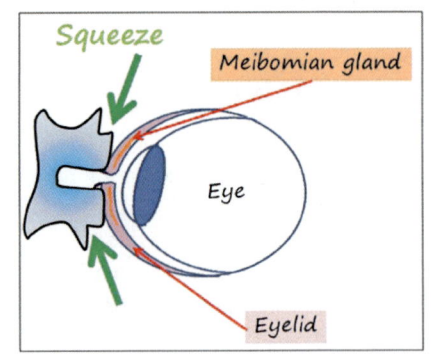

This small massage device can relieve many problems of dry eye. It is an ideal complement to the concept of "integrative facial cupping". It's called « eyepeace® ».

## REASONING

There are glands in the eyelid called "Meibomian glands". They help hydrate the cornea of the eye, protect it from toxins by producing a thin lipid layer on the surface of the eyeball. This thin lipid layer is called the "Meibum". With age, the blinking of the eye produced by the eyelid muscles is less effective. This blinking normally produces a massage of the Meibomian glands. Less Meibum weakens the eye; it is drier, more susceptible to infections and inflammation of the conjunctiva. As a result, many older people complain of having dry eyes. They often have itchy eyes with significant visual discomfort due to poor drainage of Meibomian glands. To do this, health practitioners have opted for several methods such as the small plastic massage device that we recommend (despite its price that seems high), see photos above. All gentle methods of "vibrating" the eyelid are welcome to compensate for the lack of strength of the palpebral muscles and lack of blinking of the eye. Even by massaging a simple toothbrush in the vertical direction can help drain, it's up to you to test... In the end, it is an important complement to cupping facial. You can also use small suction cups with the lowest possible suction pressure to try to "stimulate" these glands.

The medical profession has developed a massage device (lipiflow®) to heat and massage these glands. The result is guaranteed for several weeks. This will have an effect on the vitality of your face, your eyes and the comfort of your sight that will improve.

# REFERENCES

Some references that served to write this book.

**About Face-lifting protocols and cupping**

- Alghoul M, Codner M. A., Retaining Ligaments of the Face: Review of Anatomy and Clinical Applications, Aesthetic Surgery Journal, n°33, 2013.
- Disant F., Chirurgie plastique esthétique de la face et du cou, volume 2, chapitre 2, p. 36-45, 2012.
- Massry G.G, Azizzadeh B, Periorbital Fat Grafting, Facial plast chir, 2013. DOI http://dx.doi.org/10.1055/s-0033-1333842.
- Dzifa S. Kpodzo and coll, Malar Mounds and Festoons (review), Aesthetic Surgery Journal 2014, Vol. 34.
- El Sayed S.M., Mahmoud S.H. *and coll*. Methods of Wet Cupping Therapy (Al-Hijamah): In Light of Modern Medicine and Prophetic Medicine, Altern Integ Med 2013. http://dx.doi.org/10.4172/2327-5162.1000111
- Peter Moortgat P. *and coll.* The physical and physiological effects of vacuum massage on the different skin layers, Burns & Trauma, 2016.
- Tham L.M., Cupping: From a biomechanical perspective, Journal of biomechanics, 2005.
- Chirali I. Z., Traditional Chinese Medicine Cupping Therapy (2014).

https://www.amazon.fr/Ilkay-Zihni-Chirali/e/B001H6OC4Q/ref=ntt_dp_epwbk_0

**About lymphatic drainage**

- Lagier A. *and Coll.,* Lymphatic drainage of skin areas of head and neck: In vivo approach by the location of the sentinel node, Morphologie, 2014. http://dx.doi.org/10.1016/j.morpho.2014.01.001
- Skobe M. and Detmar M., Structure, Function, and Molecular Control of the Skin Lymphatic System, The Society for Investigative Dermatology, 2000.
- Vodder E., Textbook of Dr. Vodder's Manual Lymph Drainage, vol. 2, 4 th edition.
- Echegoyen J.C., *and coll.* Imaging of eyelid lymphatic drainage, Saudi Journal of Ophthalmology, 2012.

**About venous drainage**

- Despeissse M. A., la veine jugulaire externe, medical thesis, Nantes university, France, 2006 -2007.
- Pecheur M., lésions ophtalmologiques d'origine dentaires, odontology thesis, Henri Poincaré Nancy university, France, 2004.
- Mage C., Variations anatomiques de la vascularisation veineuse de la face et applications cliniques aux lambeaux et à la transplantation faciale, medical thesis, Bordeaux university, France, 2016.
- Dandekar F., et coll., Periorbital edema secondary to positive airway pressure therapy. 2015. Hindawi Publishing Corporation. Case Reports in Ophthalmological Medicine: Volume 2015.
http://dx.doi.org/10.1155/2015/126501

**About olive oil**

- Vytis Čižinauskas *and coll.*, Skin Penetration Enhancement by Natural Oils for Dihydroquercetin Delivery, Molecules 2017.
http://dx.doi.org/10.3390/molecules22091536

**About Meibomian glands**

- Dominick L Opitz D.L. *and coll.,* Diagnosis and management of meibomian gland dysfunction: optometrists' perspective, clinical optometry , 2015

# INTEGRATIVE FACIAL CUPPING

For health practitioners, beauticians or for all...
This book is practical and accessible with explanatory diagrams.

It is a simple and effective technique. The action of the suction cups acts on the different depths of the skin, muscles, and fascia. All vascular and nerve structures are stimulated. The cupping facial will have a manual lymphatic drainage (MLD) effect.

The cupping facial of this book is not based on Chinese medicine. It is based on the anatomical knowledge of the muscles and lifting concepts. By its physiological effect, cupping facial provides many reliefs.

**The first part,** insists on lymphatic drainage. It wants to be autonomous and practical for anyone with little anatomical knowledge.

    *Try the Venus-Star Protocol!!*

**The second part,** is a deepening of the knowledge of the first part on lymphatic drainage. There will also be close links between the lymphatic system and the venous system.

**The third part,** is an application of suction cups for the rejuvenation and treatment of facial wrinkles. Three protocols will be presented in relation to the notions of the mechanical properties of the skin and the aging of the face.

    *Try three protocols of rejuvenation!!*

**The fourth part,** explains three tips or methods that are included in the concept of integrative facial cupping. The face is a structure plated on a hollow sphere. So cleaning the mouth, nasal cavities, massage of the Meibomian glands are techniques that are included in this concept.

    *Try the concept of INTEGRATIVE FACIAL CUPPING!!*

So the keywords of facial cupping are drainage, lifting, muscle release and toning! The cupping facial takes care of the whole face and the surrounding areas (face, neck and low-necked). **FIRST EDITION**

Made in the USA
Las Vegas, NV
04 August 2022